the baby bump

the baby bump

100s of secrets to
surviving those
9 long months

Carley Roney

and the editors of TheBump.com

CHRONICLE BOOKS

SAN FRANCISCO

Library of Congress Cataloging-in-Publication
Data available.
ISBN-978-0-8118-7694-0

Manufactured in China

Design by Liza Aelion, Kelly Crook, Dawn Camner
Cover photos, from top:
E.D. Austin Photography;
Nicole Hill/Getty Images;
Stockfood; Burazin/Getty Images
Cover illustration by
LULU*/CWC International, Inc.
Back cover: Davies+Starr

10 9 8 7 6 5 4 3

Chronicle Books LLC
680 Second Street
San Francisco, CA 94107

www.chroniclebooks.com

The ideas, procedures, and suggestions contained in this
book are not intended as health care or other professional
advice, diagnosis, or a substitute for consulting with your
health care professional. Every baby is different and circumstances vary, so you should consult your own physician and use
your own common sense. The author and publisher offer no
warranties or guarantees, expressed or implied, in the com-
pleteness or advisability of the information contained in this
book for your particular situation, and disclaim any liability
arising from its use.

Contents

week-by-week fetal development

week 5 →
Baby is starting to form major organs, like the heart, kidneys, liver, and stomach, the nervous, circulatory, and digestive systems.

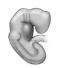

week 6 ————
As blood starts to circulate, baby's starting to develop eyes, ears, a nose, cheeks, and a chin.

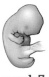

week 7 →
With joints starting to form, baby is developing arms and legs.

mom at 1 week

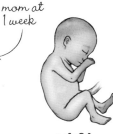

week 24 ————
As fat starts to pack on, skin is becoming more opaque and, thanks to the formation of small capillaries, it's taking on a pink glow.

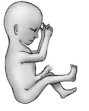

week 22 ←————
Settling into sleep cycles, baby is sleeping 12 to 14 hours a day.

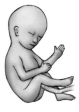

week 20 ————
Each day, baby is gulping down several ounces of amniotic fluid for nutrition and to practice swallowing—and those taste buds actually work.

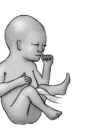

week 26 →
Baby's getting her immune system ready for life outside the womb by soaking up antibodies.

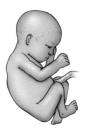

week 28 ————
Her skin is still pretty wrinkly (one by-product of living in amniotic fluid) but will smooth out as fat continues to deposit.

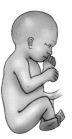

week 31 →
Baby's going through major brain and nerve development. Her irises now react to light, and all five senses work.

week 8
Continuing to straighten in the trunk, baby can move those little arms, legs, and (slightly webbed) fingers and toes.

week 9
The little embryo is now officially a fetus and a Doppler ultrasound device may be able to pick up the beating heart.

week 10
Arm joints are working as bones and cartilage are forming, and vital organs are starting to function.

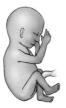

week 18
Baby has become amazingly mobile as she yawns, hiccups, rolls, twists, kicks, punches, sucks, and swallows.

week 16
Tiny bones are forming in the ears and eyebrows, and lashes and hair are starting to fill in.

week 13
While the intestines move from the umbilical cord to the fetus' tummy, baby is developing teeth and vocal cords.

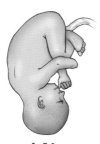

week 34
Baby can recognize and react to simple songs and may even remember them after birth. Less cute news: She now pees about a pint each day.

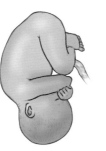

week 37
Your full-term (yay!) baby is gaining about half an ounce a day and is getting her first sticky poop (aka meconium) ready.

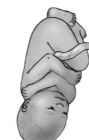

week 39
Baby's brain is still developing rapidly, and by now she's able to flex her limbs. Her nails also might start to extend past her fingertips.

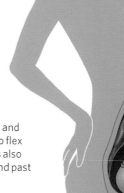

mom at 40 weeks

chapter 1

month

i'm pregnant!

one

your first big clue might be a missed period, but pregnancy... well, that starts with sex. Of course you know that, but here's a middle school bio-refresher: You have ovaries. Your ovaries have eggs. Usually, one egg pops out each month (roughly 12 to 16 days after the start of your last period), and lives for about 24 hours, meandering its way through your fallopian tube until it reaches your uterus. If you did the deed within the last few days (sperm can live for 3 to 5 days and hang out until the egg arrives) and the sperm and egg hook up, exchange genetic material, and set up shop, congrats—you're pregnant!

your to-do list

- Take a pregnancy test
- Make your first appointment with your OB
- Start eating more healthfully

Find your due date and which trimester you're in at TheBump.com/duedate

what you're in for...

"

I JUST PEED FOR THE TENTH TIME TODAY—AND IT'S NOT EVEN LUNCHTIME YET.

I think I'm getting the flu.

youch! my boobs hurt!

UGH. I FEEL LIKE MY PERIOD WILL START ANY SECOND.

umm...I was supposed to get my period on Thursday...

food sounds disgusting.

OMG—THERE'S A LINE!

I'M SOOO TIRED.

I'm feeling really bitchy.

"

on your mind...

▌ I'm pregnant?

"What's the difference between pregnancy tests? Which should I use?"

There are tons of brands and test types to choose from, ranging from $1 to around $20. And, no matter which one you get, they're all testing the same thing—your levels of a hormone called hCG. So, once your egg has been fertilized, traveled down a fallopian tube to your uterus, and dug itself a little home (aka implanted) in the uterine wall, the placenta will start cooking up hCG and dumping it into your bloodstream. Some of that hCG gets passed in your urine, too. And, that's how a pregnancy test detects it. The main difference among all these different

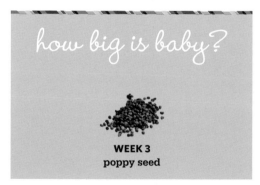

how big is baby?

WEEK 3
poppy seed

tests is how they collect your pee and show your results. Believe it or not, you have a few options.

PEE-ON-A-STICK TESTS These are without a doubt the most common tests, (maybe even the only ones you'd heard of before). They have a plastic stick with a display window and a flexible white strip sticking out one end. They all pretty much work the same way:

You pee on the strip for about 5 seconds and then wait for the results to show. Of course, be sure to read the package insert for details, but generally you're looking for a line, a plus sign, or a certain color. There's a pretty strict timeline for seeing the accurate results. So don't get impatient. Pee. Walk away for awhile and come back. Don't just stare at the stick for 15 minutes straight.

PEE-IN-A-CUP TESTS After peeing in a cup, you'll either dip a test strip in the urine or place small drops of urine onto a test that comes in a small plastic tray. Again, check out the directions for time limits and what sort of symbol means you're knocked up. There are one-step tests, where you pee in a cup, and the results show up on the side of the cup.

DIGITAL TESTS These tests are generally more expensive, but can be a sanity-saver, since the results are unmistakable. You pee on a sturdier stick, and in a few minutes the words "PREGNANT" or "NOT PREGNANT" show up on a little screen.

No matter what kind of test you end up using, the ideal time to take it is first thing in the morning—and at least a week after you were expecting your period.

"How likely would this result be a false positive?"

Did you read and follow all of the directions on the test, and check the results within the recommended time frame? And did the results look like the instructions said they would? If so—congrats!—chances are very, very slim that you aren't pregnant.

That's not to say it doesn't happen. If you miscarried or had an abortion in the past 8 weeks, have received a fertility drug that contains hCG, or have a tumor that secretes hCG, then the hormone could show up in your pee without you being pregnant. It's also not totally unheard of for a test to be defective or to give false results past its expiration date. (Take two different brands of tests if you're suspicious about your results.)

If you are testing early (especially if it's before you've had time to miss a period), there's also the possibility that the fertilized egg could implant, grow big enough to put hCG in your system, and then simply stop developing (usually because something's wrong with its chromosomes). This is called a "chemical pregnancy" and is actually super-common (it happens to over 30 percent of all fertilized eggs), but most women don't even notice. If this happened, you'd still get your period as usual (well, maybe a little bit heavier and a day or two later).

It's also possible you're seeing what's known in mom circles as an "evaporation line." Yeah, it had to get more complicated. Basically, this is when you look close and see the strip of stuff on the test that is meant to turn a color (usually pink or blue) when hCG is detected. But instead of some pretty pink or blue, you see a grayish line or what looks like a dent where the line should be. Here's the deal: If the line doesn't turn the exact

> For home pregnancy tests, I'd go for the digital ones. You can't misread them and don't need to hold the stick under different lighting to see the line. *KRISTA555*

color mentioned in the instructions (yes, again with the instructions—it never stops!), it's not positive. Similarly, if a line—of any hue—pops up after the time period specified (usually 10 minutes), it doesn't count either. Sorry for the let down.

"What if the positive line that shows up on my pregnancy test is super-faint?"
Ever hear the phrase "You can't be a little pregnant?" Apply that here. The reality is, pregnancy tests show whether or not you have hCG in your pee—they don't test how much. What this means is that if you see the line and it's the color it's supposed to be, it doesn't matter how faint or dark it seems. You're pregnant. Don't make yourself crazy second-guessing the results because you think the line isn't bold enough.

"How long should we wait before telling our family and friends we're pregnant?"
This one's totally up to the two of you. Some couples prefer to wait to share the news until the risk of miscarriage drops— when they see a heartbeat on the sonogram (at 6 to 8 weeks), hear a heartbeat with a fetal Doppler (10 to 12 weeks), or at the end of the first trimester (12 weeks). Others choose to spill the beans as soon as they test positive, rationalizing that the people they'd tell would be their network of support if anything were to go wrong.

month 1

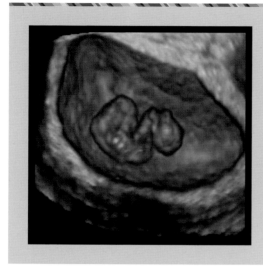

what baby's up to

- **dividing (and then redividing over and over) into identical cells**
- **digging a home in the uterine wall**
- **splitting into the embryo and placenta**
- **creating an amniotic sac and fluid**
- **forming into a tiny tadpole-like creature**

◗ at the ob's office

"So, when is my due date?"

We—and most of our doctor friends—start tallying your progress from the first day of your last period, and add 40 weeks to that date. This means counting those first couple of weeks before you actually got pregnant. Wondering why we don't just count from the day you conceived? It's hard to say exactly when that was. The best guesstimate is that you ovulated—and started this crazy journey—on about the fourteenth day of your last menstrual cycle.

This means when you say you're "4 weeks pregnant," your baby is only 2 weeks in the making. (The length of time after conception is sometimes called the "gestational age." So when you're 8 weeks, your baby's gestational age is 6 weeks.) If you don't have a due date yet, check out the predictor on page 18.

"How do I figure out what week I'm in?"

Think of it like this: When you turn one year old, you just finished your first year and entered your second year. So, when you turn 8 weeks, you'll begin your ninth week.

"Now that I know I'm pregnant, how often do I see the OB?"

Go ahead and make the call once you've had a positive pregnancy test, but all doctors are different when it comes to the timing of that first visit. Some will bring you on in, just to confirm the pregnancy (i.e., take another pregnancy test—usually just like the one you took at home). Others will schedule your first prenatal appointment for a few weeks down the line. (Lots of moms we know have started seeing the OB around week 8, others have gotten in around week 6, and some have waited until 10 or 12 weeks.)

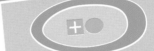

"what should I do after a positive test?"

Run for the hills! No, seriously—now's the time for celebration. If your partner wasn't there to read the test with you, share the big news and take some time to let it sink in (for both of you). If you aren't taking prenatal vitamins, now's the time to start—or at least begin a daily folic acid regimen. (It's proven to reduce the chances of neural tube defects like spina bifida if taken before conception and while pregnant.) You can also go ahead and call your OB or midwife to set up an appointment, but they might not want to see you until 6, 8, or even 12 weeks after the first day of your last menstrual period. Start taking extra-good care of yourself: eat healthy, drink lots of water, get enough rest, and stay active.

If your pregnancy is believed to be high risk—especially if you've had a few early-pregnancy losses or have a blood clotting disorder—your OB may want to have you come in earlier to keep a closer watch.

After that, your appointment schedule will vary depending on your physician, your risk level, and your (and baby's) health, but you can generally expect something like this:

4 TO 28 WEEKS One visit per month (every 4 weeks)

28 TO 36 WEEKS Two visits per month (every 2 to 3 weeks)

36 WEEKS One visit per week

are African American, have a family history of fraternal (not identical) twins, are obese or very tall, or if fertility treatments helped you to conceive. Here are some of the things that a doctor looks for:

- You're gaining weight very quickly early in your pregnancy
- Your uterus is larger than expected
- Your morning sickness is flat-out awful
- The Doppler picks up more than one heartbeat
- You get abnormal results on your multiple marker screening

If any of these things occur, your OB may decide to schedule you to get an ultrasound to confirm any extra babies. That's the only way to really tell for sure.

in your head

"How would I know if I were having a miscarriage?"

It's normal to worry, but remember that most pregnancies end with a healthy, happy baby. If you do experience a miscarriage, though, the first sign is usually vaginal bleeding. (There are other reasons for bleeding too, so don't panic. Just call your OB.) Other signs include pelvic cramps, abdominal pain, and lower back pain. It's pretty tough to self-diagnose, so talk to your doctor about any symptoms that have you feeling nervous.

"Am I carrying twins? How can I tell?"

Wondering if there's more than one little bun in your oven? You're more likely to be pregnant with multiples if you are over 30,

"So, what's the difference between identical and fraternal twins?"

With identical twins, one egg is fertilized, and then it splits into two zygotes, each of which develops into a baby. These little ones are truly two of a kind—they have the same genes, making them look just alike. They usually share a placenta too, and are pretty much always the same sex. Your chances of having identical twins has nothing to do with your age, race, or family history.

Fraternal twins are more common. They come from separate eggs that are fertilized by two separate sperm. They tend to have their own placenta, can be either sex, and come out looking about as much alike as any other (non-twin) siblings. But yeah, you can still put them in matching outfits if you want.

what's your due date?

There's no way to know for sure your delivery date. Here's how to get an idea: Simply find the first day of your last menstrual period (LMP) on this chart. Then look at the estimated date of delivery (EDD) directly below it.

LMP jan
1	2	3	4	5	6	7	8	9	10	11	12	13	14	15	16	17	18	19	20	21	22	23	24	25	26	27	28	29	30	31

EDD oct/nov
| 8 | 9 | 10 | 11 | 12 | 13 | 14 | 15 | 16 | 17 | 18 | 19 | 20 | 21 | 22 | 23 | 24 | 25 | 26 | 27 | 28 | 29 | 30 | 31 | 1 | 2 | 3 | 4 | 5 | 6 | 7 |

LMP feb
| 1 | 2 | 3 | 4 | 5 | 6 | 7 | 8 | 9 | 10 | 11 | 12 | 13 | 14 | 15 | 16 | 17 | 18 | 19 | 20 | 21 | 22 | 23 | 24 | 25 | 26 | 27 | 28 |

EDD nov/dec
| 8 | 9 | 10 | 11 | 12 | 13 | 14 | 15 | 16 | 17 | 18 | 19 | 20 | 21 | 22 | 23 | 24 | 25 | 26 | 27 | 28 | 29 | 30 | 1 | 2 | 3 | 4 | 5 |

LMP mar
| 1 | 2 | 3 | 4 | 5 | 6 | 7 | 8 | 9 | 10 | 11 | 12 | 13 | 14 | 15 | 16 | 17 | 18 | 19 | 20 | 21 | 22 | 23 | 24 | 25 | 26 | 27 | 28 | 29 | 30 | 31 |

EDD dec/jan
| 8 | 9 | 10 | 11 | 12 | 13 | 14 | 15 | 16 | 17 | 18 | 19 | 20 | 21 | 22 | 23 | 24 | 25 | 26 | 27 | 28 | 29 | 30 | 31 | 1 | 2 | 3 | 4 | 5 | 6 | 7 |

LMP apr
| 1 | 2 | 3 | 4 | 5 | 6 | 7 | 8 | 9 | 10 | 11 | 12 | 13 | 14 | 15 | 16 | 17 | 18 | 19 | 20 | 21 | 22 | 23 | 24 | 25 | 26 | 27 | 28 | 29 | 30 |

EDD jan/feb
| 8 | 9 | 10 | 11 | 12 | 13 | 14 | 15 | 16 | 17 | 18 | 19 | 20 | 21 | 22 | 23 | 24 | 25 | 26 | 27 | 28 | 29 | 30 | 31 | 1 | 2 | 3 | 4 | 5 | 6 |

LMP may
| 1 | 2 | 3 | 4 | 5 | 6 | 7 | 8 | 9 | 10 | 11 | 12 | 13 | 14 | 15 | 16 | 17 | 18 | 19 | 20 | 21 | 22 | 23 | 24 | 25 | 26 | 27 | 28 | 29 | 30 | 31 |

EDD feb/mar
| 8 | 9 | 10 | 11 | 12 | 13 | 14 | 15 | 16 | 17 | 18 | 19 | 20 | 21 | 22 | 23 | 24 | 25 | 26 | 27 | 28 | 1 | 2 | 3 | 4 | 5 | 6 | 7 | 8 | 9 | 10 |

LMP june
| 1 | 2 | 3 | 4 | 5 | 6 | 7 | 8 | 9 | 10 | 11 | 12 | 13 | 14 | 15 | 16 | 17 | 18 | 19 | 20 | 21 | 22 | 23 | 24 | 25 | 26 | 27 | 28 | 29 | 30 |

EDD mar/apr
| 8 | 9 | 10 | 11 | 12 | 13 | 14 | 15 | 16 | 17 | 18 | 19 | 20 | 21 | 22 | 23 | 24 | 25 | 26 | 27 | 28 | 29 | 30 | 31 | 1 | 2 | 3 | 4 | 5 | 6 |

LMP july
| 1 | 2 | 3 | 4 | 5 | 6 | 7 | 8 | 9 | 10 | 11 | 12 | 13 | 14 | 15 | 16 | 17 | 18 | 19 | 20 | 21 | 22 | 23 | 24 | 25 | 26 | 27 | 28 | 29 | 30 | 31 |

EDD apr/may
| 8 | 9 | 10 | 11 | 12 | 13 | 14 | 15 | 16 | 17 | 18 | 19 | 20 | 21 | 22 | 23 | 24 | 25 | 26 | 27 | 28 | 29 | 30 | 1 | 2 | 3 | 4 | 5 | 6 | 7 | 8 |

LMP aug
| 1 | 2 | 3 | 4 | 5 | 6 | 7 | 8 | 9 | 10 | 11 | 12 | 13 | 14 | 15 | 16 | 17 | 18 | 19 | 20 | 21 | 22 | 23 | 24 | 25 | 26 | 27 | 28 | 29 | 30 | 31 |

EDD may/june
| 8 | 9 | 10 | 11 | 12 | 13 | 14 | 15 | 16 | 17 | 18 | 19 | 20 | 21 | 22 | 23 | 24 | 25 | 26 | 27 | 28 | 29 | 30 | 31 | 1 | 2 | 3 | 4 | 5 | 6 | 7 |

LMP sep
| 1 | 2 | 3 | 4 | 5 | 6 | 7 | 8 | 9 | 10 | 11 | 12 | 13 | 14 | 15 | 16 | 17 | 18 | 19 | 20 | 21 | 22 | 23 | 24 | 25 | 26 | 27 | 28 | 29 | 30 |

EDD june/july
| 8 | 9 | 10 | 11 | 12 | 13 | 14 | 15 | 16 | 17 | 18 | 19 | 20 | 21 | 22 | 23 | 24 | 25 | 26 | 27 | 28 | 29 | 30 | 1 | 2 | 3 | 4 | 5 | 6 | 7 |

LMP oct
| 1 | 2 | 3 | 4 | 5 | 6 | 7 | 8 | 9 | 10 | 11 | 12 | 13 | 14 | 15 | 16 | 17 | 18 | 19 | 20 | 21 | 22 | 23 | 24 | 25 | 26 | 27 | 28 | 29 | 30 | 31 |

EDD july/aug
| 8 | 9 | 10 | 11 | 12 | 13 | 14 | 15 | 16 | 17 | 18 | 19 | 20 | 21 | 22 | 23 | 24 | 25 | 26 | 27 | 28 | 29 | 30 | 31 | 1 | 2 | 3 | 4 | 5 | 6 | 7 |

LMP nov
| 1 | 2 | 3 | 4 | 5 | 6 | 7 | 8 | 9 | 10 | 11 | 12 | 13 | 14 | 15 | 16 | 17 | 18 | 19 | 20 | 21 | 22 | 23 | 24 | 25 | 26 | 27 | 28 | 29 | 30 |

EDD aug/sep
| 8 | 9 | 10 | 11 | 12 | 13 | 14 | 15 | 16 | 17 | 18 | 19 | 20 | 21 | 22 | 23 | 24 | 25 | 26 | 27 | 28 | 29 | 30 | 31 | 1 | 2 | 3 | 4 | 5 | 6 |

LMP dec
| 1 | 2 | 3 | 4 | 5 | 6 | 7 | 8 | 9 | 10 | 11 | 12 | 13 | 14 | 15 | 16 | 17 | 18 | 19 | 20 | 21 | 22 | 23 | 24 | 25 | 26 | 27 | 28 | 29 | 30 | 31 |

EDD sep/oct
| 8 | 9 | 10 | 11 | 12 | 13 | 14 | 15 | 16 | 17 | 18 | 19 | 20 | 21 | 22 | 23 | 24 | 25 | 26 | 27 | 28 | 29 | 30 | 31 | 1 | 2 | 3 | 4 | 5 | 6 | 7 | 8 |

What about triplets and other multiples? Well, they can come from one egg splitting bunches of times, from bunches of eggs being fertilized, or a combo of the two. (So if you were say, carrying sextuplets, some could be fraternal and others identical.)

is it normal?

"Is it normal to feel not ready?"

In short, yes. In fact, it would be much weirder if you felt ready. Parenthood is a big deal. Take a deep breath, relax, and remember that billions of women have been in your shoes. Your life is about to change, but you'll be fine.

"I suddenly can't sleep! Is this because I'm pregnant?"

Probably. Between the excitement, shock, and hormones, there's no wonder you aren't getting much rest. (Lots of women complain of this in the early weeks of pregnancy.) There's no magic solution, but revamping your sleeping environment might help a bit. Start with making the room darker—try blackout liners or heavy drapes. (For a more temporary solution, you could tape up black garbage bags with painter's tape. Ugly, but

GREAT DEBATE

on antidepressants?

meds worth the risk

"The question isn't if you should take them but if you want to feel well or ill. If somebody was on heart meds, no one would tell her to stop taking them. But, for some reason, we see antidepressants as being optional. Not taking your meds leaves you at high risk of a relapse during pregnancy. The risks for baby having withdrawal are low, and all of the symptoms are mild and treatable."

Dr. Gail Robinson, CPsych, FRCPC, MD

the danger is great

"A recent review on the safety and effectiveness of antidepressants points out that newborns whose mothers used antidepressants during pregnancy have increased respiratory distress rates, feeding difficulties, and low birth weight due (in part) to baby's withdrawal. The review notes that first-trimester use may potentially lead to birth defects as well."

Dr. Kathleen Kendall-Tackett, PhD, IBCLC

Get more drug facts at **TheBump.com/meds**

effective.) Also consider lowering the temp, which helps your bodily functions slow down somewhat, making it easier to rest. The ideal temperature is 68 to 72 degrees Fahrenheit. Stick a thermometer in your room to double-check it—your thermostat only measures the temp at its own location.

"Should I be alarmed if I feel cramping?"
Lots of moms have period-like cramps in early pregnancy. As long as the sensations are mild, you (and baby) are probably just fine. If your cramping is severe, accompanied by bleeding, lasts more than a couple of days, or you just really want to get checked out, go ahead and call your OB.

"What about spotting? When should I worry about it?"
If it's the week or two after you conceived, the spotting could be implantation bleeding. This happens when your little fertilized egg starts burrowing into your uterus, and can appear as light spotting for anywhere from a few hours to a few days.

Or, since your cervix is über-sensitive right now, you might notice some bleeding after sex. If this happens, wait to have sex again until you've spoken with your OB. (Sex is considered completely safe and there's simply no reason to stop doing the deed just because you're pregnant. This is just a precaution.) Bleeding can also be a sign of infection in your pelvic cavity or urinary tract, or may simply be a result of the increased blood flow to your cervix.

Still, call your OB to discuss any bleeding or spotting. It's probably nothing to worry about, but it could also be a sign of ectopic pregnancy, molar pregnancy, or miscarriage.

is it safe?

"Is it really bad that I had four drinks—before I knew I was pregnant?"
Chances are good that you did no harm—tons of us have been in your shoes and had very healthy babies. But, now that you know you're pregnant cut out alcoholic drinks. There's a risk of Fetal Alcohol Syndrome, which can cause abnormal facial features, growth problems, and developmental and various learning disabilities.

"I heard that I shouldn't change my cat's litter box—really?"
Yes, really. (If nobody else will do the job, wear sturdy rubber gloves and just be extra-cautious not to touch the kitty poop.) Cats are known to carry a parasite called *Toxoplasma gondii*, which can put you at risk for an infection called *toxoplasmosis*. This may cross through the placenta and cause serious problems with your fetus. Our advice: (Nicely) ask your partner to suck it up for the next 9 months and clean kitty's litter box. It's also worth noting that gardening and eating raw meat puts you at risk for toxoplasmosis as well, so wear your gloves and skip the rare steaks. And, as always, wash your hands!

"how can I be sure I'm eating the things baby needs?"

Besides the 300 or so extra calories, you'll need your vitamins and minerals. Here's what you need and how to get it.

zinc

HOW MUCH 11 μg per day
WHY Zinc is linked to a lowered risk of preterm delivery, low birth weight, and prolonged labor. It prevents intrauterine growth retardation as well.
TRY Baked beans are a great choice; you'll get 1.8 μg for each half-cup serving.

folic acid

HOW MUCH 600 μg per day
WHY Even before you get pregnant, you should start increasing this one. Doing so cuts your risk of birth defects.
TRY No midnight cravings for spinach or asparagus? Try an orange for 50 μg a pop.

beta carotene

HOW MUCH 7,700 IU per day
WHY This improves skin and vision. Plus, it recharges the immune system (you really don't want to get hit with a sinus infection now!). It's also crucial for proper cell and gene development.
TRY Sweet potatoes deliver 50,000 IU in one cup!

calcium

HOW MUCH 1,000 mg per day
WHY Getting enough calcium can reduce the severity and lower the overall risk of preeclampsia, low birth weight, and preterm delivery.
TRY Yogurt has 450 mg per cup—double milk!

protein

HOW MUCH 60 to 70 g per day
WHY Your body needs a lot more protein now to help the fetus grow and ensure that baby's hormones and muscles develop properly.
TRY A lean beef or chicken burger yields 30 g—half your daily requirement!

DHA

HOW MUCH 450 mg per day
WHY Higher levels of DHA in newborns correspond to higher birth weight. It's also associated with a higher IQ, more advanced motor skills, and fewer emotional and neurological problems later.
TRY A 4-oz. serving of salmon packs a punch with 130 mg.

iron

HOW MUCH 27 mg per day
WHY Not enough can impair baby's growth and increase the risk of hypertension, eclampsia, preterm delivery, and low birth weight.
TRY A bowl of fortified cereal, at 10 mg, provides more than a serving of beef!

vitamin D

HOW MUCH 200 IU per day
WHY It helps increase blood circulation in the placenta and aids in calcium absorption.
TRY Fortified orange juice provides 50 IU per cup, so be sure to drink up!

▌the day-to-day

"When will I start showing?"

As with everything else, this is different for everyone. Your fetus is pretty tiny in the first few months, so other people won't be able to see much—if any—change in your belly. If this is your first pregnancy, it could be a long while before strangers are asking when you're due. If it's not your first pregnancy, you'll start to show much faster.

By about 12 weeks, when the top of the uterus has grown up and out of the pelvic cavity, you'll probably be able to feel it just above the pubic bone. This significant change usually signals the beginning of your visible baby bump . . . meaning, time to start browsing the maternity racks!

"I keep forgetting to take my prenatal vitamins. Is this bad? How can I get into a daily routine?"

It's even more important to get into the swing of taking your vitamins every day once you know that you're pregnant. You need the extra boost of folic acid, calcium, and iron even if you're generally a pretty healthy eater. To jump-start the habit, keep the vitamins next to your toothbrush—you know you'll brush your teeth at least twice a day, so even if you forget the pill in the morning, you'll get another shot at remembering at night. You should also carry some in your purse at all times. That way, when you remember to take them midway through your drive to work, you don't have to head all the way back home or skip them altogether.

real moms uncensored

on sharing the news . . .

"I made a onesie for my 7-month-old niece that said, 'I'm getting a cousin!'" *jesnbrent*

"When we called my husband's parents, we said, "We're calling because we wanted to tell you we're making you something . . . Grandparents!" *SeattleMermaid*

"My husband gathered us all into a group and took pictures. So it went, 'say cheese . . .' with one camera, 'say cheese . . .' with the next, and finally 'say xyz's pregnant' with his own camera. Everyone said it and then laughed . . . but then it set in, and we were able to capture everyone's reaction forever!" *RunAway*

"what exactly is in a prenatal vitamin?"

folic acid
600 μg
Prepregnancy, you need 400 μg, but up it to 600 μg to prevent birth defects.

calcium
300 mg
You'll be well on your way to your goal of 1,000 mg of calcium daily. (Yes, ice cream counts.)

iron
30 mg
Pregnancy means a 50 percent increase in blood flow. Pop 27 mg of iron a day (double the usual).

you need to keep taking this after you're pregnant

vitamin a
770 μg
Required for vision and cellular growth

vitamin c
85 mg
Aids in absorbing iron

vitamin e
15 mg
Helps heal skin irritations

thiamin
1.4 mg
Involved in both nerve and muscle function

vitamin b6
1.9 mg
Synthesizes serotonin

vitamin d
200 IU
Assists in calcium absorption—think of the two of these as partners

copper
2 mg
Helps the body to absorb iron

zinc
11 to 12 mg
Keeps you healthy

vitamin b12
2.6 μg
Helps to maintain healthy nerves and red blood cells

vitamin e
15 mg
Helps heal skin

riboflavin
1.4 mg
Needed for healthy cell function, growth, and energy

dha/omega-3
450 mg
Assists in brain development; other pills for this exist

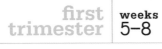

chapter 2

month

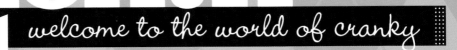

welcome to the world of cranky

two

even though you probably just got the good news, you're well over a month into pregnancy! We know it seems weird but the first 2 weeks were kind of freebies. Hang onto that feeling of excitement from the first few weeks—you'll need the pick-me-up when you start feeling like crap, right about . . . now. When you're totally annoyed for no reason and your head is about to hit your desk, remember the important part: YOU'RE PREGNANT!!! It will make you feel better (and is a pretty convenient excuse) when you can't make it through a whole hour of your favorite TV show without falling asleep (never mind trying to start a movie) or why you completely snapped when [fill in the blank].

your to-do list

- Schedule a prenatal checkup

- Get the lowdown on what you can and can't do now

- Go to your first OB appointment

Create your personalized pregnancy checklist at TheBump.com/checklist

what you're in for...

"

STAY AWAY FROM ME RIGHT NOW. I'M FEELING REALLY BITCHY.

I just peed for the tenth time and it isn't even lunchtime yet.

my areolas are dark and bumpy.

I HAVE A SECRET.

ALL OF MY SHIRTS ARE STARTING TO GET TIGHT.

I need TUMS. Now. (Hello, heartburn.)

cravings!!!

Now that the shock has worn off, I'm really excited!

UM, THERE'S SOMETHING WEIRD IN MY PANTIES. IS THIS NORMAL?

my boobs are killing!

I'm bloated and constipated!

I'M SOOOO TIRED.

I feel like I'm going to puke.

"

on your mind...

▌at the ob's office

"What, exactly, is going to happen at my first OB appointment?"

Your first trip usually includes extra poking and prodding around. Expect to give a full medical history and to have a full physical (pelvic exam, breast exam, urine test, pap smear, blood work)—even if you recently had your yearly GYN checkup. You'll also get lots of questions about your partner's family history, so bring him if you can!

Here's a breakdown of what else to expect during that first appointment:

GENETIC TESTING COUNSELING Your OB will talk about genetic testing and warning signs to watch for. It's routine—don't be alarmed.

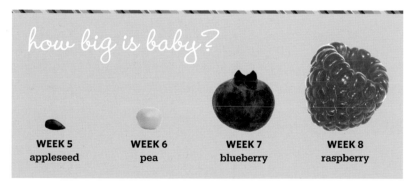

how big is baby?

WEEK 5 — appleseed
WEEK 6 — pea
WEEK 7 — blueberry
WEEK 8 — raspberry

GETTING A DUE DATE The OB will give you an estimated (now, we said *estimated*!) due date.

ULTRASOUND EXAM You may need to have an ultrasound to confirm that everything looks A-okay so far. (Quick vocab lesson: Ultrasound is the name of the procedure; the sonogram is the image that's created.)

This is also the time to ask questions and talk about all the lifestyle changes and the long list of no-nos now that you're pregnant. Based on your health and risk factors, you and your OB will work out a schedule for the rest of your appointments. The usual time frame is a visit every 4 weeks from your first visit to week 28; your appointments will pick up to every 2 to 3 weeks from weeks 28 to 36. After that, you'll see your OB each week until baby is born.

"What will an early ultrasound be like? How much will I really see?"

This early in the game, your uterus is still way down behind your pelvic bone, so you can't see much with an external ultrasound machine. That means your practitioner needs a more direct route. A transvaginal ultrasound probe (it looks kind of like a dildo and will even wear a condom) is inserted into your vagina (sounds freaky but doesn't hurt). The sound waves it emits form an image of your insides which appears on the screen for you to see. At this point, baby will look like a small, white jelly bean. Ask the technician to point out the gestational sac, yolk sac, and fetal pole (the first evidence of an embryo). And the best part: You may even be able to to see the bright, fast flutter of a heart. Oh, and don't forget to ask for a photo or two to take home!

checklist

"what questions should I ask at my first OB appointment?"

Get in the habit of keeping a pen and paper handy and jotting down questions as they come to mind. (You'll be amazed by how many you think of—and even more surprised at the havoc pregnancy wreaks on your memory.) Here are a few to get you started.

○ How much weight should I gain?

○ Do I have an increased risk of any complications or conditions?

○ What screenings do I need? Why? When will I have them?

○ What kind of diet should I follow?

○ Should I be doing any particular kind of exercise? Can I continue my workout regimen for now?

○ Are there any restrictions on sex during my pregnancy?

○ Is it okay to travel while I'm pregnant?

○ What over-the-counter meds are safe, and in what amount? Which ones should I avoid?

○ Are the prescription meds I'm currently taking safe? If not, what can I take or do instead?

○ Which prenatal vitamin do you recommend?

○ Which prenatal classes do you recommend?

○ What symptoms should I expect before my next visit and what should I do about them?

○ Do you rotate with other doctors in your office, or will I see you every visit? What about when I'm ready to deliver? Will you be in the delivery room or might it be someone else?

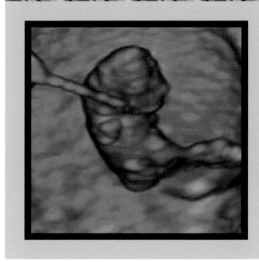

what baby's up to

- heart, brain, muscles, and bones are starting to develop
- arms and leg buds begin to form
- notches form where fingers and toes will sprout
- spinal cord is growing
- nostrils and eyes start forming
- baby's embryonic tail is gone
- arms grow longer and bend at elbows

"Are blurry and itchy eyes just another pregnancy symptom?"

Once again, blame it on the hormones. They're also making your eyes red, itchy, and sensitive to light. And the same swelling you feel in your breasts and ankles gets to your eyes as well—it's particularly troublesome if you wear contacts. Try to limit the time you spend wearing them and take them out before sleeping. Blurred or distorted vision may be a sign of a more serious condition, like high blood pressure or diabetes, so call your OB right away. Also check with her before using any eye medications.

"What are beta levels and what do they measure?"

Let's start at the very beginning. When baby first begins growing in your belly (aka uterus), your body starts producing a hormone called hCG, or human chorionic gonadotropin. (There's more on this on page 13.) This hCG stuff is sometimes called the "pregnancy hormone"—it happens to be the same one a pregnancy test screens for in your urine. It takes more than a week (typically around 11 to 14 days) after conception for enough hCG to show up in your pee. If your OB measures your "beta hCG" levels, it means she's checking to see just how much hCG is running through your blood. Any hCG level above 25 mIU/ml is considered to be positive for pregnancy, but your doctor may want to check your beta hCG levels for other reasons as well, including to determine if your pregnancy is progressing the way an average one does. (In about 85 percent of normal pregnancies, hCG levels double every 48 to 72 hours until they drop down and level off after around 8 to 11 weeks.)

"My uterus is backwards. Will this make delivery more difficult?"

What you have is called a tilted uterus. All it means is that while the average woman's uterus is tilted to the front, yours is titled the other way. It's not that uncommon, either: 15 to 20 percent of women have the same thing. During pregnancy, it will most likely tip into the normal position by week 12 or 13. If it doesn't readjust, you'll know because it will feel like you have a urinary tract infection. You'll feel pressure, and when you go to the bathroom, it will feel like you still have to pee, even though nothing more is coming out. If you have these symptoms, call your OB. As far as labor is concerned, it shouldn't make a difference. (Some people worry about being able to conceive with a tilted uterus, but that's not an issue. The sperm can get to the egg just as easily. Keep in mind that sometimes a tilted uterus can result from a more serious issue, like endometriosis.)

in your head

"It seems like so much can go wrong. How can I know my baby is okay?"

Welcome to parenthood. You're going to worry about your baby for the rest of your life. Literally. So you may as well get used to it now. The truth is, you *can't* know that baby's okay in there. You won't know he's okay with the baby-sitter either. Or at college. Yes, there is stuff that can go wrong. But, there's a much better chance that everything will be just fine and you're on your way to having a healthy little mini-me (or -he). The best thing you can do right now is focus on staying healthy and following your doctor's recommendations. Our advice: Try to stay positive, don't read the scary stuff without a good reason (like if your doctor tells you that you're at risk for something specific), and ban yourself from all of those tragic stories on the Internet. After all, this is a time when you should be celebrating—not stressing.

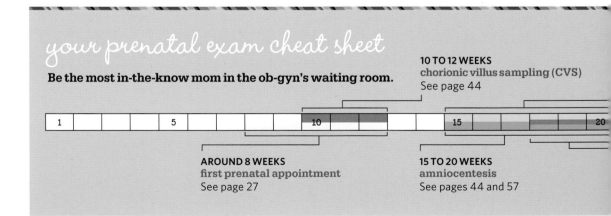

your prenatal exam cheat sheet

Be the most in-the-know mom in the ob-gyn's waiting room.

10 TO 12 WEEKS
chorionic villus sampling (CVS)
See page 44

| 1 | | | | 5 | | | | | 10 | | | | | 15 | | | | | 20 |

AROUND 8 WEEKS
first prenatal appointment
See page 27

15 TO 20 WEEKS
amniocentesis
See pages 44 and 57

"What should I do to get my finances and other important things in order before baby arrives?"

These are important questions, and now is exactly the right time to start thinking about them. (Don't panic, you're not a slacker.) Here's a quick checklist:

HEALTH INSURANCE If you don't have it, get it. Already covered? Read up on your policy so you know exactly what it covers and what it doesn't. This may also be a good time to see what you can deduct from your flexible spending account if you have one—prenatal vitamins and loads of other necessities may be game under your plan.

DISABILITY INSURANCE If you don't have it, you can't get it . . . but your partner can.

LIFE INSURANCE It's not pleasant to think about, but it is important.

SAVINGS PLAN Figure out how much you need to sock away, not just for the birth itself, but really for the next 18-plus years.

MATERNITY LEAVE Bone up on your employer's policy now, and start budgeting.

ESTATE PLANNING You may already have a 401(k), but now's a good time to update the beneficiaries if you want. If you don't have a will, talk to a lawyer about drawing up a document. (Yep, another unpleasant topic.) It's also the time to name a guardian for baby—you know, just in case.

"My partner is trying so hard to help me, but it's annoying. What can I do?"

We're sure you can think of one or two . . . or maybe one hundred things he could do that wouldn't be annoying at all, like taking over bill-paying or making you sweet potatoes (hello, cravings!). What you're feeling is totally normal. Thank your hormones, lack of sleep, or just stress, but mamas-to-be can seem downright scary. Tell your husband not to take your mood swings personally. Show him the cool, crazy pictures in your

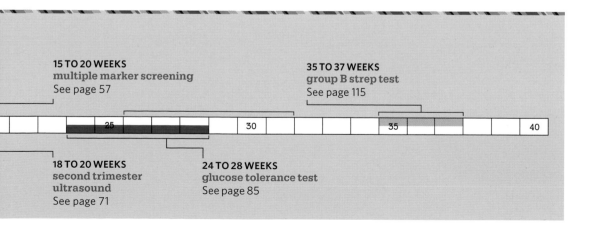

15 TO 20 WEEKS
multiple marker screening
See page 57

35 TO 37 WEEKS
group B strep test
See page 115

18 TO 20 WEEKS
second trimester ultrasound
See page 71

24 TO 28 WEEKS
glucose tolerance test
See page 85

pregnancy books, like the one illustrating that baby has grown from the size of a poppy seed to a raspberry (see page 27)! And make sure to have fun together when you're not feeling bitchy. Try a new restaurant, see a movie . . . live it up before baby starts to revamp your social calendar.

"I'm sick and sluggish (and I've had to come in late a few times), but I don't want to tell my boss about my pregnancy yet."

It does seem cruel that most women feel their worst during the first 12 weeks when you're trying to keep the news (and your nausea) hush-hush. Until you announce the good news (most people wait until 12 weeks just to be certain everything is okay), there's no milking it for (well-deserved) sympathy. And it's tough to come up with reasons for why you're acting so drained. Here are a few excuses you can try out (not to encourage trickery or anything . . .):

FOR THE SLEEPIES

- I'm fighting a nasty cold and just feel completely wiped out.
- Man, this (yawn) night class I'm taking is really getting to me.
- This kind of weather makes me so sleepy.
- This cold medicine really knocks me out.
- My coffeemaker broke this morning.
- Or put a book on sleep apnea on your desk.

FOR THE LATENESS

- I had to wait for the cable guy/plumber/ electrician.
- Arg! I locked myself out of the house again!

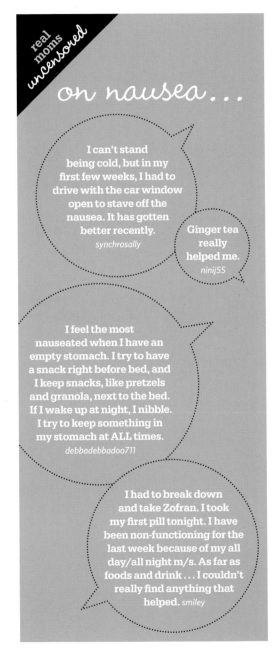

real moms uncensored

on nausea . . .

I can't stand being cold, but in my first few weeks, I had to drive with the car window open to stave off the nausea. It has gotten better recently. *synchrosally*

Ginger tea **really** helped me. *ninij55*

I feel the most nauseated when I have an empty stomach. I try to have a snack right before bed, and I keep snacks, like pretzels and granola, next to the bed. If I wake up at night, I nibble. I try to keep something in my stomach at ALL times. *debbadebbadoo711*

I had to break down and take Zofran. I took my first pill tonight. I have been non-functioning for the last week because of my all day/all night m/s. As far as foods and drink . . . I couldn't really find anything that helped. *smiley*

- My husband and I are sharing a car while the other one's in the shop. I apologize that it's made me late a few times!
- The traffic's getting really ridiculous— I've got to find a new route to work.
- I can't believe I accidentally set my alarm clock for 7 P.M. instead of A.M.!

is it normal?

"Why do I have a superhuman sense of smell? When will it go back to normal?"
Crazy, isn't it? You find out you're pregnant, and suddenly you can smell the garbage on the curb of the house three doors down. Like with most of your symptoms, hormones are to blame. This is often the worst during the first trimester (as if your nausea needed a boost) and tends to let up (at least a little) as your pregnancy progresses. Explain to your partner why he may want to take up cooking and trash duty for the next month or two, and try to surround yourself with stuff that doesn't reek (try ginger, lemon, or mint scented candles or oils).

"I've lost weight since finding out I was pregnant. That doesn't seem right."
You're growing another person and yet the scale is slipping—weird, huh? Don't worry: It happens to lots of women in the first trimester. Baby doesn't weigh much yet, and morning sickness and a puny appetite can often suck a couple of pounds away. You could also see a bit of a drop if you're eating more healthfully than before you found out the big news. Most women gain only 2 to 5 pounds in the first trimester anyway, so you won't be that far behind. Just make sure that you're taking in enough nutrients and staying hydrated, and you'll see the scale going up (and up, and up) in no time. And, as always, talk to your OB about any concerns.

"I've definitely noticed the mood swing thing. How can I balance myself out?"
Yes, hormones are partly to blame, but this time, they aren't the only culprits. Whether the pregnancy was planned or not, whether it's your first child or your fifth, having a baby is life-changing and can make you anxious and worried (totally normal). Will the baby be healthy? Can I afford it? How long will I feel sick? Will I be a good parent? With all this to think about, it's no wonder you're acting a little nuts. So how can you pull yourself together? Begin with eating healthy food and small, frequent meals, as drops in blood sugar levels can exacerbate mood swings. Exercise is also key. Try prenatal yoga to relax, and walk when you can. Besides that, get lots of rest and remember to set aside time for yourself. Enlist your partner for a shoulder rub or take a warm (not hot) bath.

> Now, every little thing makes me cry. Can't find something to wear? Tears. Something sweet/touching/sad on TV? Tears. Really tired? Tears. *Mrs._F*

If your mood swings are really getting out of control, consider couples counsling and/or stress-reduction classes. Even if you don't do counseling, it's super-important to get your partner involved. The more he understands what you're feeling (and has methods to help), the better for both of you. And don't forget to call on friends and family for support.

PS: If you think this may be more than just average mood swings, speak up. Also let your provider know if you've suffered from anxiety or depression and if you've needed meds to treat these issues in the past. She'll be able to recommend what's safe during pregnancy.

"The nausea is killing me! Is there anything that helps?"

Some women get morning sickness (okay, more like all-day sickness) much worse than others. There isn't a magic cure, but there are plenty of things you can try. For starters, don't starve yourself. While eating may sound gross, an empty stomach and low blood sugar can actually trigger nausea. Snack on mini meals throughout the day, opting for tummy-friendly food, like carbs and yogurt. Steer clear of greasy and spicy foods, which can make nausea worse. Some women swear by saltines. Keep a pack on

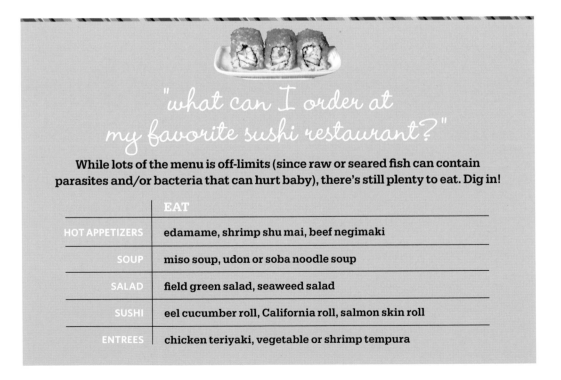

"what can I order at my favorite sushi restaurant?"

While lots of the menu is off-limits (since raw or seared fish can contain parasites and/or bacteria that can hurt baby), there's still plenty to eat. Dig in!

	EAT
HOT APPETIZERS	edamame, shrimp shu mai, beef negimaki
SOUP	miso soup, udon or soba noodle soup
SALAD	field green salad, seaweed salad
SUSHI	eel cucumber roll, California roll, salmon skin roll
ENTREES	chicken teriyaki, vegetable or shrimp tempura

your night stand for nighttime sickness, and stash a bag of them in your desk drawer for midday nausea. Ginger (as in ginger ale and ginger candy) is another excellent option. It has a long history of soothing tummies, and studies have shown that 250 mg taken up to four times daily can help (check with your OB first). Vitamin B6 has been proven to reduce queasiness too—ask your OB if you can take 25 mg tablets up to four times a day. Another secret moms swear by is sour candies. Keep a few on hand during the day. You can even slip on an accupressure band (found at most drugstores) which combats nausea by stimulating acupressure points. People use it for seasickness or car sickness. Finally, keep from getting dehydrated (a nausea trigger) by sipping water and eating hydrating foods, like Popsicles and fruit. If all else fails, check with your doctor about over-the-counter or prescription medications. If you're losing lots of weight or aren't able to keep anything down, seek help asap— it could signal a more serious condition.

"I'm not sick and my boobs aren't sore. Should I worry?"

Nope, it simply means you're lucky. Some moms have more obvious symptoms, from morning sickness to constipation, than others. Don't worry—a lack of symptoms doesn't mean anything is wrong with you or baby. Enjoy feeling normal while it lasts! Oh, and you might want to pretend to feel at least a little bit crappy around other pregnant women just so they don't hate you.

❚ is it safe to?

"Is it okay to have sex? What about as I get farther along?"

If you've got the energy, go right ahead. As long as everything is normal and everyone's healthy, sex is safe from that first positive home pregnancy test right up until your water breaks. If you're at particular risk for preterm labor or miscarriage, or if you notice unusual pain, discharge, or bleeding post-sex, your OB may recommend some precautions or limits. Even if your pregnancy is perfectly normal, warn your partner to never blow air directly into your vagina. In rare cases, this can lead to an air embolism fatal to both you and baby. (Weird but true.) And, of course, make sure you know your partner's sexual history and that he's been tested for STDs and HIV. (Yes, you learned this in seventh grade . . . but it's just that important.)

"Should I be concerned about drinking from plastic bottles?"

There has been concern that exposure to Bisphenol A, or BPA, in extremely high doses may cause miscarriage and birth defects. But the effects are noted with exposures that are more than 400 times greater than you'd experience in daily life. If you're worried, ask your doctor what she considers safe.

"I want to keep exercising, but is there anything I shouldn't do?"

Most doctors will clear you to keep up with just about any exercise you were doing before you got knocked up. But there are a couple of exceptions to this rule: contact sports (no tackle football) and ones that risk falls (like downhill skiing or horseback riding). As your uterus grows larger, you'll need to avoid lying flat on your back, but for now you're good to go. Keep in mind that your heart rate is higher during pregnancy, so go heavy on the warm up and cool down. In general, be careful. Those pesky hormones will loosen up your joints and ligaments, making you klutzy.

"Is it okay to use a vibrator?"

Unless your doctor or health care provider has specifically requested that you to refrain from sexual activity because of potential complications, it should be absolutely fine to use a vibrator. Many couples enjoy having a full sexual relationship right up to the birth of their baby. And when you consider that penetrative sex involves active thrusting, the vibrator seems mild in comparison. Also, there's no reason to skip using a vibrator externally on your clitoral region, as that's a very good way to climax (however, if you have a high-risk pregnancy, check with your OB first). If you have a clean bill of health and your pregnancy is going swimmingly, you still might find that you're more satis-fied having sex the old-fashioned way or by using the vibrator internally.

"I heard I shouldn't be in a hot tub while I'm pregnant. Why?"

The problem with a hot tub (or steam room, or sauna) is that it can raise your—and baby's—core body temp too high. There's

evidence that temps over 102 degrees could lead to neural tube defects, brain damage, fetal growth restriction, and miscarriage. So nothing super-hot, please.

"Do I have to stop painting my nails?"

Manicures and pedicures have gotten a bad rap because of a certain chemical that's found in many brands of nail polish called dibutyl phthalate, or DBP. Some experts argue that it can be harmful to your fetus. Others say there's no hardcore evidence that an occasional mani/pedi is unsafe. Your best bet: Choose polish that doesn't have DBP, toluene, or formaldehyde on the ingredient list, and bring it with you to the salon.

the day-to-day

"How can I get around tipping off my friends when we go out for drinks?"

There's no bigger pregnancy giveaway than the lush who suddenly turns into Little Miss Teetotaler. So let them pour your wine and then fake sips throughout the meal (your partner can also surreptitiously drink from your glass.) Or head to the bar alone and order a mocktail. We're partial to sparkling grape juice and fruit puree or sparkling water mixed with pomegranate or cranberry juice and a squeeze of lime. If you're a beer drinker, try this trick: Order a dark bottle, take it with you to the ladies' room, empty it out, and fill it with water. Not ideal, but it works!

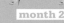

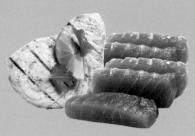

raw meat is a no-no too

month 2

"so, what can't I eat?"

Now that you're eating for two, what goes in your mouth is very important. Here's what's off-limits (or partially off-limits) and why.

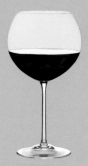

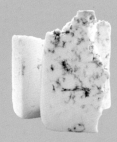

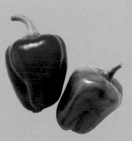

alcohol It goes into baby's bloodstream and could lead to big problems, from an increased miscarriage risk to issues related to development.

certain fish Stay away from swordfish, king mackerel, tilefish, and shark, which contain high levels of mercury. Any type of raw fish is also a no-no.

soft, unpasteurized cheese Unpasteurized types, like feta and goat cheese, can contain disease-spreading organisms that put you and baby at risk.

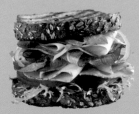

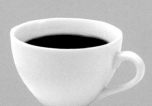

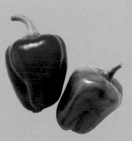

deli meat It could carry listeria, a bacterium that causes serious illness. To play it safe, reheat deli meat to at least 165 degrees before eating.

coffee The jury is out on caffeine, but most OBs recommend limiting intake (no more than one or two caffeinated beverages a day) or cutting it out completely.

unwashed produce Make sure you clean fruits and veggies to rid them of bacteria.

"my boobs are huge...is it maternity bra time or should I just go up a size?"

Yes, your boobs are changing. When to buy a maternity bra and what to do in the interim? Check out our bra map.

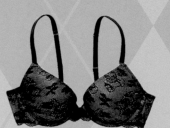

MONTHS 1 TO 3
your regular bra
You can probably get away with your regular bra for the first couple of months. But be realistic and prepare to go up a size soon.

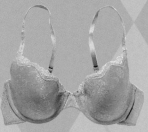

MONTHS 4 TO 6
cheap bigger bra
Hold off on a maternity bra and instead go up in band and cup size. The key: Think cheap. You won't be wearing this bra for long.

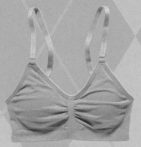

MONTHS 7 TO 9
maternity bra
Give in and go for it. A maternity bra gives you major support, especially along your sides, which can get really sore now. Invest in two and rotate them.

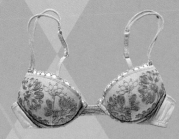

the cups just unhook and fold down

POSTBABY
nursing bra
Your goal: support and easy access. Skip the underwire—it puts too much pressure on your breasts and can cause clogged ducts.

POSTBABY
new sexy bra
Your boobs won't be the same—even if your size is back to normal. Now's the time to splurge on at least one sexy new bra.

"Is pregnancy brain real?"

Fortunately (or unfortunately, depending on how you look at it), there's no scientific research that proves you get flaky while pregnant. But there are still tons of mamas-to-be who say they feel more forgetful and spaced out. So what's to blame? Hormonal changes, lack of sleep, and/or not being able to stop thinking (and stressing!) about your new baby. Save your sanity by writing down everything, as well as making lists. Regular snacks and getting lots of rest will help you feel a lot more like your old self too. And be sure to take your prenatal vitamins—they contain a number of ingredients that help boost mental sharpness.

"Why am I having *crazy* dreams?"

Dreams reflect your mental state, and let's face it—you're kind of a basket case right now. Hormonal changes—specifically, progesterone and estrogen surges—also contribute to wacky dreams. And, don't forget your constant nighttime awakenings. Dreams come during deep REM sleep, and when you wake during this stage, it's much easier to remember a dream. So why are you dreaming about rainforests and oceans . . . and talking animals . . . and sex (not just with your spouse) . . . and tall buildings? These common themes represent emotions and anxieties about your changing body, the person growing inside you, and your evolving relationship with your mate. Think of it as your subconscious way of working through stress and those heavy emotions.

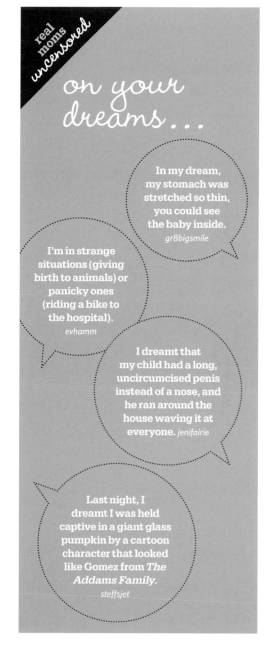

real moms uncensored

on your dreams . . .

In my dream, my stomach was stretched so thin, you could see the baby inside. *gr8bigsmile*

I'm in strange situations (giving birth to animals) or panicky ones (riding a bike to the hospital). *evhamm*

I dreamt that my child had a long, uncircumcised penis instead of a nose, and he ran around the house waving it at everyone. *jenifairie*

Last night, I dreamt I was held captive in a giant glass pumpkin by a cartoon character that looked like Gomez from *The Addams Family*. *steffsjet*

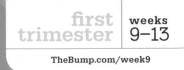

chapter 3

month
three

there's a light at the end of the tunnel

good news! Right now, you're probably still feeling a little out of it (okay, maybe a lot), you'll be turning the corner in just a few weeks. Wahoo! Plus, there's something huge to look forward to: This is the month when your OB will (probably) start listening to baby's heartbeat at each visit—there's no cooler sound for a mama-to-be than the thump-thumping you're going to hear (don't be freaked out that it's fast; that's totally normal). So take the leftover nasties in stride and look forward to an increasing appetite, an increasing waistline, and (hopefully) a decreasing sense of having to throw up at any given moment.

your to-do list

- Hear heartbeat with Doppler

- Buy a bigger bra

- Start shopping for maternity clothes

- Decide when and how to spread the word

▶ **Get the lowdown on building your maternity clothes wardrobe at** TheBump.com/matclothes

what you're in for...

"Weird—that sounds like a horse galloping.

I'M PEEING CONSTANTLY.

I've got bluish veins showing up under the skin on my boobs.

Another zit? And this one's on my back!

my boobs are getting huge!

I need TUMS. Now. (Hello, heartburn.)

I have *extra* discharge in my panties.

I'M CONSTANTLY HUNGRY.

gas!

I'm feeling cranky, tired, and nauseous."

on your mind...

▌ at the ob's office

"When will I get to hear the heartbeat? What does the heart rate mean?"

Your OB will probably listen for the heartbeat with a Doppler ultrasound device around week 12. (Some of our mom friends have had doctors try a little earlier, but usually not before week 10.) Anything between 110 and 160 beats per minute is considered "normal." And though we've heard many a grandma claim that the heart rate can reveal baby's sex, scientists say no way. In fact, the heart rate changes a lot—even baby wiggling around can speed it up. (But if you want to play along for fun, the old wives' tale is that girls have faster heartbeats.)

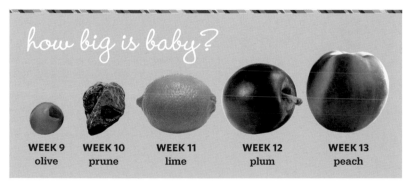

how big is baby?

WEEK 9	WEEK 10	WEEK 11	WEEK 12	WEEK 13
olive	prune	lime	plum	peach

"What's an NT scan? I've heard of it but don't know if I need one."

The nuchal translucency screening (or NT scan) is a special ultrasound, given between weeks 11 and 14, that checks the volume of the clear, fluid-filled space in the back of baby's growing neck. If there is more fluid than normal, it could be an early warning sign for Down syndrome, trisomy 18, and other chromosomal disorders, as well as congenital heart defects. This scan is often done in combination with a serum test to check certain hormone levels (PAAP-A and beta-hCG) in your blood. (You might hear the full deal referred to as your "first trimester screening.") Like other screenings, you won't get any definites—only an alert for potential risks. If the test finds abnormal results, they'll offer further tests, like amniocentesis (which is done around weeks 15 to 18).

"How do I know which trimester I'm in?"

Ah, this is a tricky one! As you've probably noticed, the answer will depend on who you ask. Different OBs use different markers to determine the start and end dates of each trimester. We know, this makes things confusing—especially when people ask what trimester you're in! Some doctors divide it into equal thirds, others break it up into three chunks of 13 weeks with an extra week at the end, for a grand total of 40 weeks. You'll probably come across a couple of other methods out there, but this is the most common breakdown:

FIRST TRIMESTER first day of your last menstrual period (LMP) through week 13
SECOND TRIMESTER weeks 14 through 27
THIRD TRIMESTER week 28 through labor

month 3

"I'm going to have prenatal diagnostic testing done. How do I decide between CVS and amniocentesis?"

Both have benefits. CVS (chorionic villus sampling) is done earlier, usually around weeks 11 or 12, which means putting an end to your worries sooner (hopefully), or, in a worst-case scenario, you'll have more time to reflect on the results. CVS results also come back quicker than amnio's. It may be difficult to find an experienced provider to do the test, though, because fewer doctors perform CVS than amnio. But, if you're at particular risk for neural tube defects, such as spina bifida, amnio is the clear choice—CVS won't detect these. Amnio, which tends to be done around weeks 15 to 18, also allows you to postpone making your decision (to test or not to test) until after you've seen the results of your second trimester screenings.

▍in your head

"When does my chance for miscarriage drop?"

Most miscarriages occur in the first trimester and are due to chromosomal problems that happen during fertilization. Unfortunately, it's estimated that between 10 and 15 percent of pregnancies end in miscarriage, and there usually isn't any way to prevent it. While this number may seem high, look at the flip side: There's an 85 to 90 percent chance that everything will be fine. Plus, those stats

include women who miscarry so early on, they didn't even know they were pregnant. Most miscarriages involve bleeding and/or cramping. But—and this is important—if you have bleeding in your first trimester, don't panic; more than half the time, it stops and the pregnancy continues to term. In some cases, there are no warning signs until an ultrasound reveals that there's no heartbeat (this is known as a "missed miscarriage").

So, when can you stop worrying? Seeing or hearing a heartbeat means your risk is just 3 percent. And after a normal 16-weeks ultrasound, it's down to 1 percent.

"Is there any way I can tell if it's a boy or a girl before my big ultrasound?"

There's no way to be 100 percent positive, but there are a number of at-home urine tests you can pick up at the drugstore or mass-market retailers. These tests typically claims 82 to 90 percent accuracy and can be used as early as 10 weeks (6 weeks from your first missed period). That's accurate enough to be fun, but you'll still want to wait until your OB confirms baby's sex via an ultrasound at around 18 weeks or an amnio (weeks 15 to 18). Of course, you could try the Chinese Gender Chart on page 47. No guarantees, but still!

"What kind of expenses should we be prepared for when baby arrives?"

You'll be faced with lots of one-time expenses, like the nursery and all the furniture inside it. Keep in mind that you can register for many of the items including the crib and

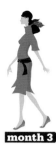

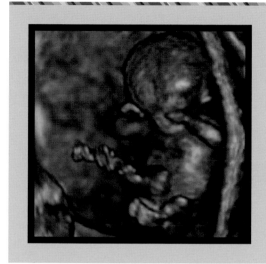

what baby's up to

- intestines begin moving from umbilical cord to baby's tummy
- graduates from "embryo" to "fetus"
- arm and leg joints start working
- fingers and toes lose webbing
- skin is see-through
- vital organs begin to function
- bones and cartilage develop
- teeth and vocal cords form
- arms and feet start to take shape (yep, even little toes and fingers!)
- hair follicles, tooth buds, nail beds form

the dresser. You also need to think about monthly expenses, like diapers, formula and food, clothes, toys, and laundry costs. Even if you just sock away $100 a month, start a savings account for baby as soon as possible.

▌ is it normal?

"I feel like I pee every five minutes! Why?"
For one thing, the hormone hCG triggers an increase in blood flow to the pelvic area, which makes your body produce more pee. At the same time, your kidneys are kicking into high gear and working more efficiently than ever, so your body gets rid of waste more quickly. And let's not forget your grow-ing uterus, which puts loads of pressure on your bladder as it gets bigger.

The good news is, this pressure lifts once the uterus rises into your abdominal cavity in the second trimester. Until then, be sure to lean forward when you pee to completely empty your bladder. This might cut back on trips to the ladies' room. And even if you're tempted, don't stop downing liquids—your body needs them to stay hydrated.

"I'm having a lot of cramping. Is there something wrong with my baby?"
Probably not. It's normal to have period-like cramping at the beginning of pregnancy (see more on page 20), but it isn't 'til a little later that abdominal cramping comes into play. It's just one of those things that happens when a baby is growing in your belly. (And growing from the size of an olive to the size of a peach, like baby is this month, is pretty significant.) Doctors call it round ligament

pain. See, your uterus is growing every day, and the muscles and ligaments supporting it are stretching to accommodate the changes. Stretching can bring some pain, especially when you change positions, cough, or are particularly active. These mild aches are normal and (sorry) may keep happening as your uterus gets bigger. For relief, scale back physical activity and avoid cramp-inducing positions. Also try a warm bath, or just stretch out and kick up your heels.

Don't worry unless the pain is severe, continual, or accompanied by bleeding or other unusual signs. If you have any of these symptoms, call your doctor right away.

"Will the heartburn be this bad for the next 6 months? Will anything help?"

In early pregnancy, progesterone helps the muscles of your uterus relax to stretch for baby, which also relaxes the valve between your esophagus and stomach. That burning you feel is literally stomach acid bubbling up from your gut. The good news is, heartburn may ease up in the second trimester. But, the bad part: That's also just about the time baby will begin to squash your digestive organs, causing the same problems. You can't really get that valve to shut again, but you might find some relief by avoiding triggers like chocolate, coffee, tea, citrus, tomato sauces, and spicy and fried foods. It also helps to sleep with your head elevated a bit, and to hold off drinking too much with meals.

Just be sure you get plenty of water an hour before and an hour after meals so you don't get dehydrated. The fact is, no matter what you do, you'll probably still feel the burn sometimes. Talk to your doctor about what meds are safe. She'll probably recommend an antacid, like TUMS, to start, or something stronger if you're especially miserable.

"What's up with all this saliva?"

Are you also super-queasy? Experts aren't sure why, but women who experience lots of nausea and vomiting also seem to complain about extra saliva. It's probably hormone related. (Plus, nausea can lessen your desire to swallow, making you stockpile your spit.) Luckily, this tends to be only a first-trimester issue—the drool should dry up a bit in coming weeks. Until then, keep hard candy or sugarless gum in your purse (they make it easier to swallow). Some say frequent mouthwash and tooth-brushing help too.

"Why am I getting awful headaches?"

Surging hormones, higher blood circulation, stress, lack of sleep, dehydration, and, hello, caffeine withdrawal can all lead to a pounding head. Luckily, the headaches should go away in your second trimester as your body adjusts to the new hormone levels. In the meantime, get plenty of sleep, exercise, eat healthily, and stay hydrated. If the pain does hit, apply a warm compress to your face or a cold compress to the back

> Sometimes my headaches get so bad that they turn into full-blown migraines. All I can do is take Tylenol and lie down in a dark, quiet room with a cold washcloth on my forehead until I manage to fall asleep.
>
> *sweetpea814*

chinese gender chart

This chart is said to be over 90 percent accurate in predicting baby's gender.
Match your age at conception to the month you did the deed!

month 3 ▶

month of conception

your age at conception

	jan	feb	mar	apr	may	jun	jul	aug	sep	oct	nov	dec
18												
19												
20												
21												
22												
23												
24												
25												
26												
27												
28												
29												
30												
31												
32												
33												
34												
35												
36												
37												
38												
39												
40												
41												
42												
43												
44												
45												

of your neck, rest in a dark room, or take a warm shower. If none of these relieve the pain, talk to your doctor about which pain medications are okay to try.

"I'm having a lot (and I mean a lot) of discharge. Is this normal?"

As long as it is clear or whitish and has, at most, a mild smell, and you aren't itching or burning, then yes—it's normal. It's called *leukorrhea*, and is made up of secretions from your cervix and vagina. You've probably seen this discharge before, but it's extra-heavy in pregnancy thanks to vamped-up estrogen production and blood flow to the vagina. You can't get rid of it, but you wouldn't want to—it's your body's natural way of expelling bacteria that could harm both you and baby.

Invest in a box of unscented panty liners and stay away from tight clothes, scented pads, douches, and any other feminine care products. Also stock up on cotton panties— they wick moisture and are best for keeping your girly bits clean and dry.

Leukorrhea usually tends to get heavier in the days just before labor hits. If you notice this happening before week 37—or if it's pink or brownish at any time during your pregnancy—give your OB a call right away. This could be a sign of preterm labor. Also get checked by your doctor if, in addition to the discharge, you're itching or burning or notice a strange smell. You may have a yeast infection.

"Help! I haven't pooped in three days!"

Yikes! Constipation is par for the course, but there are some things you can do to help move things along. Fill up on fiber (whole grains, fruits, and veggies) and drink lots (as in eight or more glasses a day) of liquids, especially water. Though you may not feel so motivated right now, exercise can help too. Whatever you do, try not to push too hard when you're trying to do your business. (It can lead to a major case of hemorrhoids.) If your system still can't get regular, ask your OB about using Colace or Metamucil. Don't take any meds or home remedies without asking—enemas, laxatives, or other methods could stimulate labor.

▌is it safe?

"I want to have sex, but my husband's afraid he'll hurt the baby. Crazy, right?"

Some guys have a tough time with the idea of pregnant sex. First, try assuring him that there is no way a penis (no matter how, um, large) can poke the baby and harm it—or hurt you. The fetus is safely tucked away in your uterus and surrounded by amniotic fluid. Plus, there's a thick mucus plug that's there to stop germs from getting inside. If he's still not buying it, bring him with you to your next OB appointment and let the doctor speak with him directly.

> I know there is absolutely no way to hurt the little one, but it freaks us both out. I'm afraid I'll start spotting afterward and just go crazy. My husband is afraid baby will see his goods and will be scarred for life!
>
> *CapeSummer21*

"how much weight am I supposed to gain?"

If your weight was in the normal range (body mass index of 18 to 25) before conception, the American College of Obstetricians and Gynecologists (ACOG) recommends that you gain 25 to 35 pounds by the time you deliver. On average, that means adding 3 to 5 pounds in the first trimester, then about a pound each week through month 8 (weight gain slows a little in the ninth month).

However, if you were underweight before you got pregnant, you should gain a little more (28 to 40 pounds). If you're overweight, try to keep it to a max of 25 pounds. No matter what your starting weight, your goal is to gain as steadily as possible. If your weight suddenly changes, especially in the third trimester, contact your doctor. This could signal a serious condition called preeclampsia.

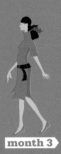

month 3

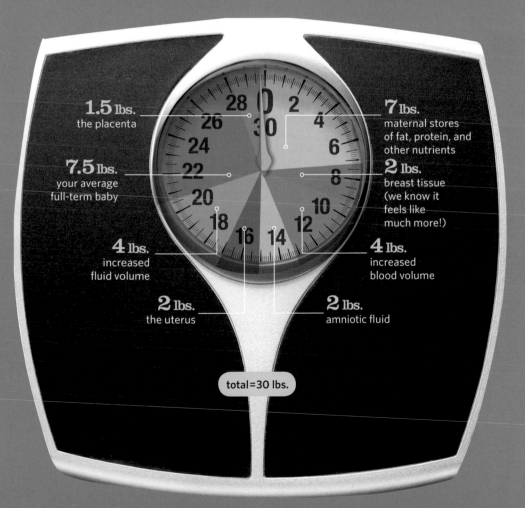

1.5 lbs. the placenta

7 lbs. maternal stores of fat, protein, and other nutrients

7.5 lbs. your average full-term baby

2 lbs. breast tissue (we know it feels like much more!)

4 lbs. increased fluid volume

4 lbs. increased blood volume

2 lbs. the uterus

2 lbs. amniotic fluid

total=30 lbs.

"I'm tempted to buy a Doppler and listen to the baby at home."
You can buy a fetal heart monitor—aka a Doppler machine—from a ton of retailers. (Google "fetal Doppler" and you'll be flooded with results.) Most of these are pretty much the same as what your OB uses, and yep, you can use them to listen for the little one. They seem to be safe for baby too—just remember you might not find the peace of mind you're after. Sometimes, it can be tough to find the fetal heartbeat, stressing out many a mama to no end. Our doctor friends have had a ton of calls from women freaked out about changes in the heart rate too. Keep in mind anything between 110 and 160 BPM is cool.

"Can I still visit the chiropractor?"
Not only can you—you should! Getting regularly adjusted while pregnant can relieve stress on your spine that comes with the weight gain. It can also prevent sciatica, the inflammation of the sciatic nerve that runs from your lower back down your legs and to your feet. Regular visits can help maintain pelvic balance as well, which is often thrown off as your belly starts to grow and your posture begins to change. In addition, studies have shown that chiropractic adjustments control nausea, prevent a potential c-section, and even reduce the amount of time some women spend in labor.

"Is it safe to dye my hair?"
No scientific study has proven whether hair color is 100 percent safe during pregnancy, but most doctors now agree that you can cover your roots and grays (with some restrictions; see below). The potential risks involve the chemicals used in dye entering your system, either through your skin or through the air you breathe. To minimize risks, consider these precautions:
• Wait until after your first trimester, when baby's vital organs are already developed.
• Choose the earliest salon appointment to minimize exposure to chemicals.
• Ask your stylist to avoid letting the dye touch your scalp.
• Go for highlights rather than permanent or semi-permanent color. Highlight solution is covered in foil and doesn't come in contact with the scalp.
• Ask your colorist about natural henna.
• Talk to your stylist about dyes with little or no ammonia or peroxide.
• If you DIY, be sure to wear gloves and work in a well-ventilated room.

"Can I take regular gym classes or can I only do prenatal ones?"
It's likely okay to keep going to your regular classes—just listen to your body and clear it with your OB. You'll need to modify some exercises as your pregnancy progresses, and some regular classes may be too tough as your belly expands. Let the instructor know you're pregnant and ask for pointers. And in general, stop doing an exercise if it doesn't feel good, if you feel nauseated, light-headed, or overheated. You should also lay off of high-impact aerobics (no kick boxing), stay

month 3

real moms uncensored
on constipation...

> I am going about every four days. It sucks. I have never in my life so freely talked about poop with my husband. *buckeybride107*

> Go straight for the prune juice. Nothing else worked for me. *dreamsicle23*

> Just be careful you don't get hemorrhoids. NOT FUN. *bottomstar*

> Remember that upping your fiber intake without upping your water intake will only make the problem **worse.** *kimilane*

off your back after the first trimester, and make sure you've got something to lean on for support during balance exercises (your center of gravity is about to undergo a major shift). Keep these tips in mind as well:

WEAR THE RIGHT GEAR Your boobs are super-sensitive right now, so find a sports bra that fits well and does its job as a supporting star.

WARM UP Those 5 minutes of easing in can mean the difference between achy calves and not—you have enough other aches right now.

DON'T GO HIGH IMPACT No jumping around or doing anything too crazy.

GET UP SLOWLY If you've been working out while lying down, like doing sit-ups, you could get light-headed. Plus, after the first trimester, you can't do exercises on your back at all.

DON'T PUSH YOURSELF TOO HARD Take breaks when you're tired.

COOL DOWN Give yourself 15 minutes.

▌the day to day

"My clothes are getting tight, but I'm not ready for maternity clothes yet. Any ideas for this in-between stage?"

Hoping to squeeze into your favorite jeans for another week or two or three? The "rubber band trick" is an old favorite of ours: For extra room around the waist, take a regular rubber band or hair elastic, loop it around your pant button, and then thread it through the button hole and loop back around the button. A big safety pin works too. Pull over a long sweater

"what staples should I have in my closet to get me through my pregnancy?"

☑ you have   ☐ you need

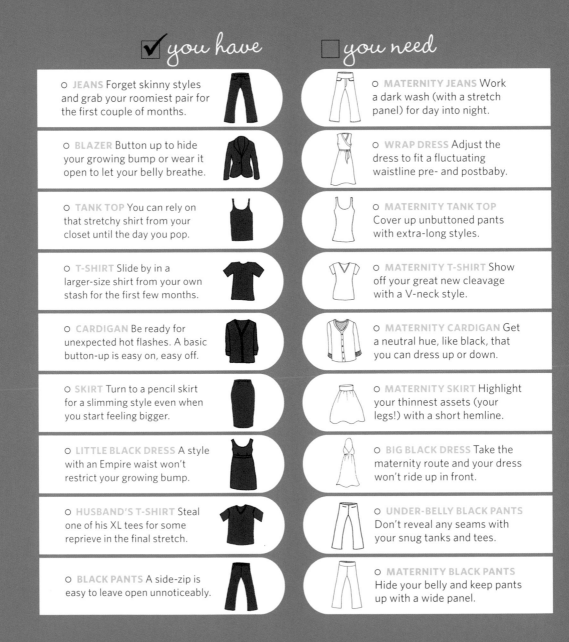

○ **JEANS** Forget skinny styles and grab your roomiest pair for the first couple of months.

○ **MATERNITY JEANS** Work a dark wash (with a stretch panel) for day into night.

○ **BLAZER** Button up to hide your growing bump or wear it open to let your belly breathe.

○ **WRAP DRESS** Adjust the dress to fit a fluctuating waistline pre- and postbaby.

○ **TANK TOP** You can rely on that stretchy shirt from your closet until the day you pop.

○ **MATERNITY TANK TOP** Cover up unbuttoned pants with extra-long styles.

○ **T-SHIRT** Slide by in a larger-size shirt from your own stash for the first few months.

○ **MATERNITY T-SHIRT** Show off your great new cleavage with a V-neck style.

○ **CARDIGAN** Be ready for unexpected hot flashes. A basic button-up is easy on, easy off.

○ **MATERNITY CARDIGAN** Get a neutral hue, like black, that you can dress up or down.

○ **SKIRT** Turn to a pencil skirt for a slimming style even when you start feeling bigger.

○ **MATERNITY SKIRT** Highlight your thinnest assets (your legs!) with a short hemline.

○ **LITTLE BLACK DRESS** A style with an Empire waist won't restrict your growing bump.

○ **BIG BLACK DRESS** Take the maternity route and your dress won't ride up in front.

○ **HUSBAND'S T-SHIRT** Steal one of his XL tees for some reprieve in the final stretch.

○ **UNDER-BELLY BLACK PANTS** Don't reveal any seams with your snug tanks and tees.

○ **BLACK PANTS** A side-zip is easy to leave open unnoticeably.

○ **MATERNITY BLACK PANTS** Hide your belly and keep pants up with a wide panel.

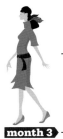

month 3

or blouse and no one will be the wiser. Or, grab a belly band. You can find some version at most maternity stores. It's essentially a tube of fabric that stretches over your belly to hold up unbuttoned bottoms or maternity jeans that are too big, support your belly as it grows, and smooth over your "outie" when it inevitably pops. As for tops, dig through your closet for pieces that give you some space. Empire waists and flowing silhouettes will conform to your expanding figure. Raid your guy's closet too, and don't be shy to ask for short-term loans from a one-size-bigger friend. (Pay it forward by offering up your own goods when a pal is pregnant.)

"I know being super-emotional is part of pregnancy, but how do I deal?"

Blame this one on the hormones! During the first few months after conception, levels of hormones, like estrogen and progesterone, change dramatically, which in turn has a significant effect on brain chemistry (that explains why you're suddenly bursting into tears during dog food commercials). For most women, moodiness is most noticeable in the first few months of pregnancy, then again in the last weeks leading up to delivery and often for a while after baby's born. If yours seem extreme or are affecting your way of life, bring it up with your doctor. She'll be able to guide you to further forms of care that are safe and effective. But rest assured that what you're feeling is totally normal. Sometimes you just have to stop and remind yourself that it's the hormones talking (or crying or screaming) and not "the real you!"

"I deserve some pampering before baby arrives, right? Any creative ideas?"

Prenatal pampering is definitely one of the biggest trends around—and rightfully so! Here are some of our favorite ways to treat yourself (and you partner) before diaper-changing and 2 A.M. feedings take over:

HIRE A BABY PLANNER They'll help you design a nursery, set up your baby registry, and even send out birth announcements when the time comes. Come on, you had a wedding planner. . . doesn't baby deserve the same treatment?

TAKE A BABYMOON With a new baby on the way, it's tough to predict the next time you and your husband will be able to get some alone time, let alone an actual getaway. That's why now is such a perfect opportunity to sneak off for a romantic just-for-two vacation. Hotels and resorts offer tons of fun packages exclusively for moms-to-be and their partners. You won't be sorry—guaranteed!

HIRE A PHOTOGRAPHER FOR MATERNITY PHOTOS At first, it may sound like the world's worst idea—pay to document your expanding belly and create a lifelong keepsake?! But trust us: Tasteful maternity photos are the perfect way to capture the innate beauty of your pregnant body and your personality.

GET A FOOD DELIVERY SERVICE It's tough enough to maintain a healthy diet when life is normal. Add the nutritional demands of pregnancy plus your never-ending to-do list, and you've got a perfectly legitimate reason to splurge. Some delivery services even have special menu plans designed specifically for pregnant women, so do your research first. And ask for a taste test before you commit long-term.

chapter 4

month

one trimester down

four

hello, second trimester! Time to pull your head out of the sand (or the toilet) and enjoy the real perks of pregnancy, like chivalry from complete strangers and a cute round tummy popping from under your shirt. Any day now, you should be gaining energy, sanity—and a whole new wardrobe! Your chance for miscarriage has dropped super-low by now, too, so go ahead and spread the big news if you've been holding out. (You'd better hurry before your swelling belly tips them off.)

your to-do list

- Start sleeping on your side

- Look into maternity leave

- Schedule your mid-pregnancy ultrasound

Download our maternity leave checklist at TheBump.com/matleave

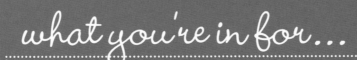

what you're in for…

" my belly feels stretched!

my bump is noticeable.

I finally have energy again.

I HAVE BLEEDING GUMS.

Wow! I think I felt a kick.

the morning sickness is gone.

I NEED NEW CLOTHES.

WHOA, I'M GAINING A LOT OF WEIGHT NOW.

"

on your mind...

▌at the ob's office

"What is a multiple marker screening? How do I know if I need one?"

It's a simple blood test that checks for an increased risk of certain conditions (Down syndrome, trisomy 18, and neural tube defects). You might also hear this called a *triple screen* or *quad screen*, depending on how many wild and crazy hormones your OB wants to measure. A triple screen looks at your levels of estriol, human chorionic gonadotropin (hCG), and alpha-fetoprotein (AFP). A quad screen also measures the hormone inhibin-A.

Talk with your OB about which screening is right for you. And remember, like other

The multiple marker screening is only accurate from weeks 15 to 20, so ask your OB about it at this month's appointment so she can set it up in the next couple of weeks.

"What happens during amniocentesis?"

Amniocentesis (often called "amnio") is a test that uses a long, thin, hollow needle to suck about an ounce of fluid from the amniotic sac (the bag of liquid surrounding baby). First, the OB will use ultrasound to find a nice pocket of fluid that isn't too close to baby or your placenta. Once she sticks you, the needle stays in from 30 seconds to a few minutes. Most moms say it doesn't hurt too bad. In the lab, baby's cells are taken from the liquid, grown in a culture for about 10 days, and then studied for chromosomal abnormalities (plus genetic disorders, if you're at risk). The

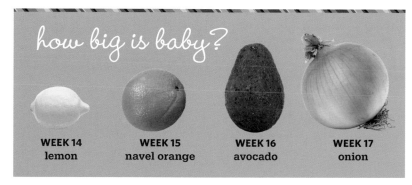

how big is baby?

WEEK 14	WEEK 15	WEEK 16	WEEK 17
lemon	navel orange	avocado	onion

month 4 ▶

screenings, you won't get any definites: Abnormal results are possible even if your baby's fine, or you may get normal results even if she does have one of the conditions. The point of a screening is simply to identify your level of risk. It's not a "yes" or "no" test. If results suggest a risk, you'll be offered CVS or amniocentesis, which can diagnose these conditions, if one does exist.

alpha-fetoprotein levels in the fluid are also measured, to help detect neural tube defects like spina bifida. If you're interested, the test is accurate at revealing baby's gender. Amnio results usually take about two weeks.

Amniocentesis does carry a slight risk of miscarriage (about 0.5 percent), so it's not a routine procedure. Your OB is more likely to suggest it if baby is at an increased risk of chromosomal or genetic defects, if earlier screenings suggest potential problems, or if you're over age 35.

If you're gearing up for amnio (it tends to be performed between weeks 15 and 20), reduce risk by checking out your provider's level of experience. If you're referred to a specialist or a testing center, ask about their procedure-related miscarriage rate and how many tests they perform yearly (look for someone who does fifty or more). Same goes for the ultrasound technician—experience reduces risk of injury and increases chances of getting a good sample on the first attempt.

When to worry: Call your OB after testing if you have severe cramping, begin leaking fluid, or develop a fever—these are all signs of possible infection or miscarriage.

in your head

"When will I feel the baby kick? And what exactly will it feel like?"

It won't be long! Most first-time moms feel movement at some point between 16 and 22 weeks. You might feel it a bit earlier in subsequent pregnancies, since you'll already know what it feels like or, if you have an anterior placenta (in front of your uterus) or are overweight, it may be a bit later than 22 weeks. Some moms feel what they call "flutters" or "bubbles." Since baby still has a ton of room to maneuver, it won't feel like real kicks or jabs just yet. Instead, it's more of a gentle sensation like a little wave, but

everyone experiences it differently. You might notice the kicking only if you're sitting or lying quietly. And don't worry too much if your pregnant friends feel kicks sooner than you do—those early kicks can be difficult to distinguish from the other weird stuff going on in your belly, like gas, and they can be pretty infrequent.

"My morning sickness is gone, I'm not so tired, and I don't feel very pregnant. How do I know this is REAL?"

Funny, isn't it? At first you wish for all the nasty symptoms to let up, and then it feels weird when they do. Luckily, feeling good doesn't make you any less pregnant. Stop worrying and try to enjoy your newfound ability to keep your eyes open (and your food down). It's normal to feel a bit strange right now, especially if you aren't showing much or feeling the baby yet. Use all that energy to start planning the nursery, or to organize your maternity leave—or your closet. Get as much as possible done and out of the way while you're feeling good.

"Will I get stretch marks? Is there any way to prevent them?"

Stretch marks pop up on the bellies, bottoms, boobs, or backs of over half of pregnant women. You probably won't see them until your skin starts expanding super-quick in month 6 or 7, and you're more likely to get them if you are carrying multiples, have a big baby, or are gaining weight especially quickly. Genetics factor in too. Did your mom or sister

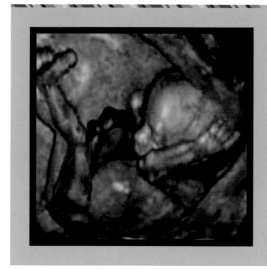

what baby's up to

- thumb sucking
- mastering the art of toe wiggling
- "breathing" amniotic fluid
- liver, kidneys, and spleen continue to develop
- lanugo (thin, downy hair) grows
- joints officially work on all four limbs
- hearing begins to develop
- eyebrows, eyelashes, hair, and taste buds form
- skeleton begins to harden
- finger (and toe!) prints form

month 4

get stretch marks? If so, you probably will too. (Sorry about that.)

There's no hard evidence that lotions, creams, or oils will actually prevent the marks, but moisturizing does seem to help protect skin's elasticity, so it's worth a shot. (These formulas also helps tame the itching that can come with stretching skin, so it's a win-win.) We know moms that swear by cocoa butter and others that flat-out love some of the fancy products you'll find at maternity shops. They all pretty much serve the same purpose. Pick one now and start massaging it in regularly to get your skin ready for the months ahead. Apply after a bath or shower while your skin is still damp to lock in the moisture.

If you do get stretch marks, don't worry—they should fade considerably in the months after you deliver. And if you're uncomfortable

with your skin later, your dermatologist can offer treatment options like prescription creams and laser therapy.

is it normal?

"I feel unattractive since gaining my pregnancy weight and I'm self-conscious about having sex with my husband. Am I crazy?"

This is totally normal. It's easy for women in general (even those who aren't pregnant) to get wrapped up in little insecurities. Multiply that by ten for you—your body is changing so much right now. It's a lot to get used to. But relax. The truth is, your guy thinks of you in a completely different way than you see yourself in the mirror. He doesn't notice every extra pound. When he looks at you he sees the whole package of the woman he loves. He probably tells you this, but he does want to be with you. So take a deep breath, remember he loves you and keep reminding yourself what a fabulous mom-to-be you are. If none of this helps, do things that will make you feel better about putting on the extra pounds (as long as your OB says its okay) like walking or taking the stairs instead of the elevator when you can.

"My friend is due 2 weeks after me and she has this cute bump. I'm barely showing! Could something be wrong?"
No—"showing" later doesn't usually have anything to do with baby's size. As long as your OB says your pregnancy is on track, there's no need to worry. (At your appointment, she'll feel the size of your uterus—it'll be about 1½ inches below your belly button by the end of the month.) Some women just pop out sooner than others. Assume this means you have stronger ab muscles than your pal (don't tell her we said that), and enjoy wearing your clothes a little longer. Before you know it, you'll be wondering how your giant belly grew overnight.

"My belly cramped and got super-hard after I had an orgasm. Should I worry?"
It's normal for your uterus to contract when you orgasm. It's always done that—now it's just a good deal bigger so you notice it a whole lot more.

This won't hurt baby, and it doesn't mean you're going into labor. Don't worry, unless the cramping is especially severe, lasts more than a few minutes, intensifies, or seems to be turning into a series of contractions. If this happens, or if you have bright-red bleeding (not just spotting), call your OB right away. It could signal a miscarriage.

"My hair's going nuts. What can I do?"
We all know women who have thick, lustrous locks during pregnancy, but some of us aren't so lucky. Hormones hit every head in a different way; dry hair may turn oily and curls may straighten. Oh, and that's just the beginning— hair might start sprouting on other parts of your body too!
You know you can't change your hormones (you would have done this weeks ago if it were an option), but you can be extra-nice to your hair and hope it reciprocates. Start with nutrition: Yogurt, fresh fruits and veggies, seeds, and whole grains are especially good for hair. Keep track of the nutrients you're taking in—dry, brittle hair that falls out easily or lightens in color might be a sign of iron, iodine, or protein deficiencies. You can also help undernourished hair by giving yourself a daily 5-minute scalp massage to stimulate circulation. Or try an at-home oil treatment (great for fighting frizz). Massage half a cup

> My hair has become so greasy and oily and I have an awful, awful dry scalp. I seriously look like I'm going through puberty again.
> *ernlei608*

"what should I ask HR about my maternity leave?"

Every company's different, and state laws differ, too. When you're ready to talk to human resources, bring these questions. And take notes!

month 4

- What is going to happen during the rest of my pregnancy?
- What kind of paid and unpaid leave is available?
- While I am on leave, is my job protected?
- What provisions are there for me to ease into coming back?
- What type of leave do I have to cover my doctor's appointments?
- Is there less strenuous work available while I am pregnant?
- What kind of policies do we have for maternity leave and bonding time?

- Am I covered by the Family and Medical Leave Act or a similar state law?
- What kind of policies do we have for short term disability?
- Does our state have a temporary disability program?
- What will happen to my job while I am gone?
- What will happen to my benefits while I am on leave?
- What policies do you have to support new parents on the job?

of warm vegetable or olive oil into your scalp and hair, and let it soak under a shower cap for half an hour or so before washing it out.

"Why are my teeth and gums so incredibly sensitive?"

It's the hormones again, and it's normal—especially in the second trimester. But talk to your OB or dentist if your gums turn bright red, feel really sore, and bleed very easily. These are symptoms of pregnancy gingivitis, which could turn into an even more serious condition called periodontitis if left untreated. (Periodontitis has been linked to premature and low birth-weight babies.)

To keep your mouth in check, brush and floss at least twice a day (including gums), avoid sweets (especially chewy ones), and up your calcium and vitamin C intake. It may also help to switch to a softer toothbrush.

Go ahead and pay a visit to your dentist early in your pregnancy—just make sure to mention your condition and avoid X-ray exposure. And, don't worry . . . your gums should return to normal soon after delivery.

❧ is it safe?

"What should I do if I get a cold? Is there any chance it can hurt the baby?"

It would be nice if pregnant women were magically shielded from sickness, but it just doesn't work that way. It's totally normal to catch a cold or two, and it's not likely to have any effect on your baby. But you do need to keep a watch on your symptoms. Some things you normally wouldn't think twice about, like a headache, can actually be a sign of complications. Let your OB know when you're not feeling well. And definitely give her a call before taking any medication—even over-the-counter ones and herbal remedies. Some medicines get the green light during pregnancy, but others can harm your baby. And there are some that are fine on their own but can be dangerous if you combine them. Many OBs will give out a list of meds that they consider safe—keep this stuck to your fridge or in another easy-to-remember place. In general, to help yourself get (and stay!) healthy, you know the drill: Take your vitamins, eat healthy, drink lots of water, and get plenty of rest.

"When should I start sleeping on my side? What if I wake up on my back?"

Most OBs recommend you start sleeping on your side right about now (after your first trimester). The left side is ideal, since this position improves blood flow throughout your body, including getting it to your baby.

The problem with lying on your back (awake or asleep) is that it shifts the weight of your growing belly onto a major vein that moves blood to the heart from your feet and legs, forcing your heart to work harder. Don't freak about it though—most doctors will tell you it's okay if you wake on your back now and then. Changing positions while you snooze is normal, and your body will

real moms uncensored

on your bump...

> I find myself putting on tighter shirts just to see if my bump looks like a bump yet.
> *MrsC08*

> It seems like I woke up one morning and I had popped overnight. Hello, bump!
> *MrsHT*

> One day it just popped out and now I am excited because I actually look pregnant and not like I have a beer gut! *greens13*

> I was at the bookstore and this woman walked up to me, put her hand on my belly and said, "I've heard pregnant women hate this, but I just can't help myself!"
> *Island_Mama81*

generally let you know if something isn't right. Still, try to train yourself to spend the night on your side. If you have trouble getting comfy, try rigging up pillows (body length and/or regular) to wedge yourself into a good spot. Some moms swear by pregnancy pillows which support your head, back, hips, and belly all at once. Just warn your mate—there may not be much room for him!

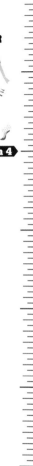

month 4

"Is it safe to eat food that's been sitting out on a buffet? How about leftovers?"

The basic rule is that if it's usually served hot, eat it hot. And if it's usually served cold, eat it cold. You're especially vulnerable to bacteria when you're pregnant, so stay away from hot or cold food that's been sitting out at room temperature for 2 hours or more. If you're at a party and want to go for seconds, reach for safe items like veggies, fruits, and bread. Dying for more mini meatballs after the 2-hour rule? It's okay to pop them in the microwave for a couple of minutes to zap any bacteria that's hanging around. Same goes for other foods that are normally served hot—a quick zap should keep you safe. As for leftovers, be sure to store them in the fridge and reheat thoroughly.

"Are there exercises I shouldn't do now that I'm in the second trimester?"

At this point you should avoid lying flat on your back for any length of time—it can reduce blood flow to baby. Otherwise, just keep listening to your body, and steering clear of contact sports and anything where you're likely to fall or get hurt. No skiing or skydiving until after delivery.

"I have a long-awaited cross-country trip planned. Is it okay to fly for so long?"
If you're having a healthy pregnancy, yes! And you should—because once baby comes, it'll be difficult just to make it to the grocery store, let alone from one coast to the other. During the flight, make sure to get up and walk around to avoid deep vein thrombosis (DVT) in which a blood clot forms deep in the vein. Pregnancy increases the risk of DVT due to your body's natural tendency to prevent excessive bleeding during childbirth. You should also drink plenty of water and other safe beverages to combat dehydration. Check with your doctor, but if you're having a normal pregnancy, most OBs say you can travel until 32 or 36 weeks. After that, you run the risk of going into labor mid-flight.

"I have a very high-pressure job. Can stress have a negative impact on my baby? If so, what can I do?"
The simple, honest answer is that stress is not good for your baby. Studies show that stress during pregnancy can lead to preterm labor and low birth weight. There's even evidence that babies who experience stress in utero are more likely to develop chronic health problems later on.

That said, stress is an inevitable part of all our lives, and only one factor among many in maintaining a healthy pregnancy. The last thing we want is for women to start stressing about the stress in their lives. With work stress, think about ways to take on a lighter load. Now is the time to start wrapping up projects, not take on new ones. After all, maternity leave is right around the corner. So start delegating and crossing things off your list. If a job-share arrangement is an option at your office, consider that as well.

If reducing your workload isn't feasible, there are plenty of tools out there to help manage the stress, including journaling, meditation, prenatal yoga, counseling, and stress-reduction classes. Even getting lost in a book or curling up with a season of your favorite TV show can help ease post-work anxiety. And don't forget to set aside some time for regular, low-impact exercise (our favorite stress-buster) and eat frequent, small, healthy meals and snacks throughout the day. The healthier your body, the better it will be able to handle the inevitable stress inducers thrown at it.

the day to day

"Do I REALLY have to drink 3 or 4 glasses of milk a day? I don't care for the stuff."
There's a loophole: This recommendation is based on your need for calcium, which you can get from lots of other foods as well. Milk just happens to be one of the most common sources. You'll need about 1,000 mg per day, which is about four servings of calcium-rich

"what are some healthy ways I can eat to get in my extra calories?"

Excellent question! An extra serving of Doritos will give you calories, but won't do baby much good. Try these (roughly) 300 calorie ideas the next time you're reaching for a mini-meal.

month 4

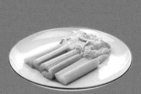

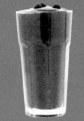

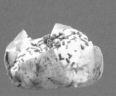

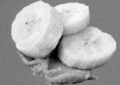

hummus scooped with your favorite assorted raw veggies, like carrots or celery

8-ounce smoothie made with your favorite mixed berries, and soy or skim milk

small baked potato topped with plain yogurt (instead of sour cream) and chives

a banana and 1 Tbl. peanut butter make it even healthier with all-natural PB

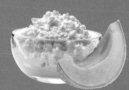

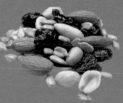

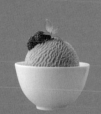

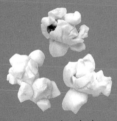

½ cup low-fat cottage cheese with one cup of fresh fruit dropped on top

dried fruit and nuts just a small handful has plenty of healthy fats and proteins

1 cup of sorbet or vanilla ice cream topped with fresh fruit

popcorn six whole cups of the air-popped kind with ¼ cup parmesan cheese

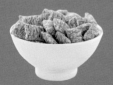

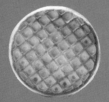

1 cup whole-grain cereal mixed with soy or skim milk for breakfast anytime

¼ cup salsa paired with two handfuls of your favorite baked tortilla chips

avocado cut ¼ of one and spread it out onto eight whole-grain crackers

whole grain waffle right out of the toaster and with peanut or almond butter on top

foods. Why so much? Well, baby's bones have to come from somewhere. In fact, if you skimp on calcium in your diet, baby will start leaching it from your bones. (Not good.) Besides milk, you can get your daily dose of calcium from cheese and yogurt, tofu, OJ, tortillas, boiled turnip greens, fortified bread, sardines, and canned salmon. Your prenatal vitamin should have at least 150 to 200 mg of calcium too, and you can always pick up an extra supplement if your diet needs a boost. Grab one that lists calcium carbonate as the main ingredient—it's easiest for your body to absorb. And check that it says "lead free." Some so-called "natural"

supplements actually contain lead, which is bad for both you and baby.

"I am so sick of water. How else can I get my liquids in?"

Water really is the best way to stay hydrated, but other things count, too. Even fruits and veggies add to the "8 cups a day" tally. (Five servings of produce = 2 servings of fluid.) And don't forget Popsicles! You may feel like you're going to float away, but don't stop drinking. Instead, think about all the great things downing a glass of H_2O can do: form amniotic fluid, produce extra blood, build new tissue, carry nutrients, help indigestion, and

---

GREAT DEBATE

alcohol during pregnancy: is a little okay?

not even a drop

"No amount of alcohol at any point during pregnancy is safe. There's a good deal of inaccurate information, even from OBs—they'll still say it's okay to drink a little bit. But we don't know that. There are no scientific studies because we can't do clinical trials on this sort of thing. A baby's brain is very susceptible to alcohol at all points in the pregnancy. And there's no way to know if there's a small amount you 'could' drink." *Dr. Susan D. Rich, MD, MPH*

sure, take a sip

"There's no data that says even one drink a day can cause fetal alcohol syndrome. Possible? Sure. But we just don't know. From a rational point of view, an occasional glass of wine is fine. Europe has produced pretty good thought leaders over the years. Einstein was a German fellow, and it's hard to imagine his mom didn't have a drink while she was pregnant." *Dr. Mary Jane Minkin, MD*

▶ Read more about drinking at **TheBump.com/alcohol**

flush out your wastes and toxins (baby's, too). Drinking lots of liquids during pregnancy can also ease constipation (and hemorrhoids), soften your skin, reduce edema, and decrease risk of urinary tract infections and preterm labor. Now, don't you want to drink up!

"I'm a vegetarian. Can I keep up my diet and still provide baby all he needs?"

Of course. The main thing to watch out for is your protein intake. But many foods besides meat are rich in protein: eggs, tofu, soy burgers, legumes (beans, chickpeas, lentils, peas), whole grains (eat with legumes for a complete protein), nuts and seeds, milk, soy milk, cheese, fruits and vegetables, and peanut butter (now you've got a good excuse to eat a spoonful straight from the jar!).

Pay special attention to other nutrients usually found in meat too, like vitamin B12, zinc, iron, omega-3 fatty acids, vitamin D, and calcium. And, of course, don't forget your prenatal vitamin!

"I need some ideas to help hide my pregnancy just a little longer."

Hiding the big news can get more difficult as your belly begins to grow, but here are a few fashion tips that might help:
- Wear black—it's the color of disguise. (You may want to keep this up postpartum, too!)
- Choose boxy layers. A suit jacket over a black top offers ideal bump coverage when you're at the office.
- Drape a scarf around your neck and knot it loosely in front to camouflage a growing

bust. The V shape it creates will draw the attention up toward your face.
- Keep eyes focused up top with red lipstick, big earrings, or a chunky necklace.

"Forget hiding it! Any ways I can look MORE pregnant?"

If you're really itching to put that new bump in the spotlight, look for maternity styles that invite eyes to focus on your midsection. The dead giveaway: anything with a sash that ties above your belly. Snug, bump-hugging tops in bright colors or patterns are a surefire way to draw attention to your middle, too. Or, if you seriously want to shout it out, grab a silly graphic T with "baby on board," "yes, I'm pregnant," or "due in February" printed across the front. (It doesn't get any more obvious than that!)

"How and when should I tell my boss that I'm pregnant?"

There's no official rule, but most women wait until the end of the first trimester when miscarriage risk is reduced. One strategy is to wait to tell her after you've completed an assignment—this sends the message that your condition hasn't impacted productivity and that you have every intention of doing your job (and doing it very well) for the rest of your pregnancy. Before you talk, outline your responsibilites and suggest ways your duties can be covered during your leave. She'll be more likely to greet the news with enthusiasm if she knows that you've got the situation under control.

month 4

chapter 5

month

bump alert

five

welcome to the fun stuff!

This month, your bump will start seriously taking shape, bringing on smiles from strangers (and hopefully no unwanted belly-pats) and a better fit to your maternity clothes. You may even be forced (poor you) to go shoe shopping as your feet grow about half a size. If you haven't felt baby's kicks yet, you will start to do so any day now, and you'll probably get a peek at her tiny profile during your mid-pregnancy ultrasound—this also means you may find out baby's gender this month, making it a good time to narrow down names, register for gifts, start shopping, and get the nursery under way.

your to-do list

- Have mid-pregnancy ultrasound

- Register for baby

- Think about the nursery setup

- Decide on (and agree on!) favorite names

▶ **Search from 1000s of fantastic names at TheBump.com/names**

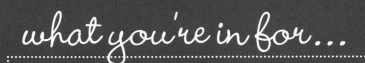

what you're in for...

"

My skin is so dry and itchy.

shoe shopping!

it's a girl!

My bump finally exceeded my boobs.

eating constantly.

is orange more of a girl color or a boy color?

WHY IS MY PULSE RACING?

WTF WAS THAT? THE BABY DEFINITELY KICKED!

my back hurts a lot.

OMG— charley horse! "

on your mind...

▌at the ob's office

"What will our big ultrasound be like?"

Your mid-pregnancy ultrasound will happen between weeks 18 and 22, and it's usually a "level two" ultrasound (meaning it's pretty detailed). Every office does it differently, but in general, it goes something like this: You lay back, the ultrasound technician glops some gel on your belly (if you're lucky, they'll warm it first), and rubs a wand-like device on your bump; then, baby's mug pops up on a screen! You may be able to watch (depends on the setup) as the tech spends a ton of time checking for fetal heartbeat, fetal location, breathing, movement, placental location and size, and amount of amniotic fluid, and taking

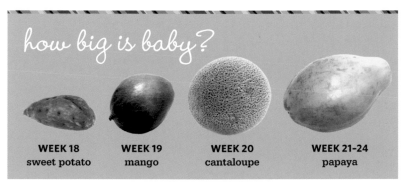

how big is baby?

WEEK 18	WEEK 19	WEEK 20	WEEK 21-24
sweet potato	mango	cantaloupe	papaya

a bunch of measurements that check for abnormalities. And—if you're interested and baby's cooperative—the technician can tell you the sex. (Let the shopping begin!)

You'll probably have a follow-up chat with your OB to discuss baby's status and you'll walk away with your first baby pic. Tip: Buddy up with the tech and she'll likely put more effort into snagging a great profile shot.

"What's placenta previa?"

Placenta previa is a rare condition where the placenta partially or totally covers the cervix. This can be dangerous when the cervix starts opening in preparation for labor, because it forces the placenta to detach, leading to bleeding. Nearly all cases of placenta previa are identified early these days, either during a routine ultrasound or when a mom-to-be complains of bright red bleeding in her second or third trimester. If you're diagnosed with placenta previa, tell any doctor you see during pregnancy, even your primary care physician. They'll want to avoid any prodding near your cervix. (If you were wondering, yes, sadly, this means sex is out too.) The good news is that your placenta may move in later months. In fact, in most cases, the placenta slides out of the way well before delivery.

Your OB will probably do a few ultrasounds to track the position of your rogue placenta. If it sticks around the cervix farther into pregnancy, you may have to be put on bed rest or given other lifestyle restrictions to avoid bleeding. One thing to note, if you've got placenta previa that continues late into your pregnancy, your OB will schedule you for a c-section before your cervix has a chance to dilate and cause trouble for either you or the baby.

month 5

"What's an anterior placenta?"

"Anterior" means "front." If you've been told you have an anterior placenta, it simply means it's located in the front of your uterus, closest to your belly instead of in the back ("posterior"), which is more common. What does this mean for you? Nothing huge, really. Amniocentesis can be a little more challenging with a placenta up front, but in general, an anterior placenta doesn't pose any serious threat to either you or baby.

"What's up with 3-D ultrasounds?"

All ultrasounds use sound waves and not radiation, to take a snapshot of your fetus. 2-D ultrasounds allow you to see a simple cross-section profile, while 3-D ultrasounds look more like a real photo, with a three-dimensional rendering of your baby's body (see the example in the What Baby's Up To box on the facing page). The image is achieved by sending sound waves at different angles and by collecting more detailed data to show depth and volume. 4-D ultrasounds take it a step further and, much like a video, collect images over time—so you will actually get to see your little one moving around in your belly in real time (making faces, kicking, sucking her thumb, the works). They are fun—and most moms want to do it at least once to sneak a peek—but don't make a monthly habit out of it.

> At my 3-D ultrasound the tech warned that baby would still look somewhat skeletal. Honestly, I think she looked beautiful. We got a great profile shot and you could already see her features. *BottomStar*

▌in your head

"What can I say when people ask me how much weight I've gained?"

Funny how people somehow think this is an appropriate question, right? If you don't feel like sharing the poundage, evade the question. Here are a few phrases that might help.
• "Oh, enough! This baby sure likes chocolate."
• "So far, so good—the doctor says I'm right on track with her expectations."
• "Not as much as I thought I would. I think the yoga classes are helping."
• "Ha. You can really tell the baby's growing, right? It's started kicking now too."

Resist the urge to dig back with, "I see you've gained weight too. How much?" Tempting, we know—but not so nice.

"Will my body ever be the same?"

No, not likely. But that's okay. Your body is an amazing thing, designed to be stretched and pulled. The skin on your middle may never be as firm, and you could wind up with stretch-mark souvenirs. But you'll probably also gain some sexy curves. Take good care of yourself now, keep it up postpartum, and you'll be somewhat back to normal. Trust us, if you exercise and stay within the advised weight-gain ranges, you'll have a much easier time toning up and dropping the "baby weight" after delivery. Don't expect to slim down overnight, though. Your body's going through 9 months of changes. It can take another 9 to 12 to get back into gear.

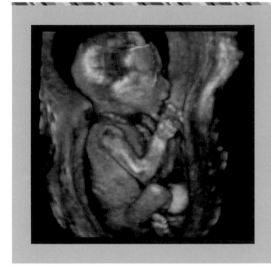

what baby's up to

- yawning and hiccupping
- flipping, twisting, and kicking
- sucking and swallowing
- creating meconium (the stuff that will fill baby's first diaper)
- vernix caseosa (greasy, white stuff) covers the skin
- genitals are fully formed
- taste buds work
- eyelids and eyebrows are well developed
- fingernails cover the fingertips

month 5

▌is it normal?

"Why is my skin itchy? And what can I do to make it stop?"

It's normal for your belly and boobs to itch like crazy as your body grows to accommodate baby. All that skin stretching is the culprit—it really dries things out. Your best bet is to dress in soft, comfy clothes and grease up with lotions, creams, or oils. Go for unscented stuff; it's less likely to irritate. Try applying them right after a shower while your skin is still damp to lock in the moisture. Colloidal oatmeal baths are also great for relieving the itchies and soothing skin. (A good thing to remember if you wind up with a rashy baby.) You can make your own if you grind the heck out of oats with a coffee grinder (essentially to powder form) and drop a couple of cups worth into a warm bath. Or just pick up some oatmeal bath from your local drugstore. And,

when you bathe or shower, remember to keep the temp at lukewarm. Hot water can have a drying effect. (Not to mention, you don't want to overheat.) If your skin starts itching all over (not just your abdomen), let your OB know. This could signal a more serious problem.

"My partner hasn't felt the baby kick. How can I help him feel it?"

Like just about everything else, this one's slightly different from woman to woman (and pregnancy to pregnancy). You may have started feeling baby dance around in there, but it usually takes a little longer for the jabs to be felt from the outside. Most moms say others are able to feel their babies kick sometime between 20 and 30 weeks. Once you start to feel baby's little knees and elbows jabbing the surface of your belly, you can give your partner a heads up on times that baby is particularly active, like just after you drink a glass of cold milk, or when you lay down at night. Cuddle up with his hand resting gently on your tummy, and sooner or later (he'll have to be patient, of course) he just may feel a little thump!

"No one told me I'd have varicose veins in my . . . vulva! Is there anything I can do?"
Your veins are working overtime right now thanks to your expanding uterus, increased blood volume, and crazy hormones. And, in the spots that are under the majority of the pressure, including your legs, vulva, and rectum (sorry) blood can accumulate. The result: swollen, or varicose, veins. So, that's the bad news, but on the bright side, aside from some throbbing here and there, they're pretty harmless and will probably disappear after delivery. To keep them under control (or prevent them in the first place), do things to improve your circulation. Prop your legs up as often as you can, exercise, avoid tight shoes, and try sleeping on your left side so your uterus doesn't press on the vena cava, a major vein on your right side (tuck a small pillow between your legs to take the pressure off your lower back though).

"Is it possible that I could have developed a third nipple from being pregnant?"
Ummm, the short answer: yes. But, it was probably there before and the changes in your breast tissue have simply made it more noticeable. Don't worry, you're not a freak—it's pretty normal, even if it seems weird.

real moms uncensored

on names . . .

I really didn't want to choose names that were popular but unfortunately, my top two girl names that I've loved since high school are in the top 20. I decided to stick with them anyway because DH likes them too.
bakeslaueabean

I think if you love the name, the popularity shouldn't matter.
monkey7106

We didn't share our name choice until after the baby was born because we didn't want to hear anyone's opinion. Of course, my MIL expressed her dislike of our "new-age name" the minute our daughter was born.
spartanmommy

❚the day to day

"It's a girl (or boy)! How should we go about sharing the news?"

It's always exciting to announce what baby's gender is! Here are a few fun ideas:

• Order a cake with pink or blue frosting inside—the first slice reveals baby's sex!

• Buy "I love Grandma" (or Grandpa) onesies in blue or pink, and give them as a gift.

• Walk in wearing a maternity T that spells it out ("It's a girl!" or "It's a boy!").

• Order custom fortune cookies with the big news hidden inside.

• Invite everyone over to watch a video of the ultrasound and guess the sex. After, have one guest open a gift that reveals the truth.

"How can I track my belly as it grows?"

Your doctor keeps track of the growth of your uterus by measuring from the top of your pubic bone to the top of the fundus of your uterus. However, it isn't so accurate to try at home. The OB is more experienced in feeling the difference between the top of your uterus and your other insides. Plus, other bump-watching methods are way more fun! Try taking a picture of yourself in profile every day or once a week (stand in the same spot and wear tight clothing). Then, combine the pictures into a flip book or digital slideshow, and you won't believe how much your body is morphing! (This makes a great keepsake of your pregnancy.)

Some moms also like to track belly growth by measuring their used-to-be waistlines and then recording weekly measurements in the baby book or a pregnancy journal. You'll rack up a lot of inches in the weeks to come!

"What size clothes should I buy for my newborn baby?"

Aside from your OB's estimations (which can sometimes be way off), there's no way to know what clothing size baby will fit into on day one. Many a new mom ends up with piles of barely worn newborn clothes, and many others bring baby home to a wardrobe entirely stocked with too-big clothes. Even if you think you're carrying a linebacker, buy a few newborn-sized outfits (usually fits babies who are 8 to 12 pounds)—just leave the tags on all but a few of them. Be sure to stock up on several 0 to 3 outfits too, in case baby outgrows the newborn duds super-quick. And if you wind up with a teeny baby? You can always have Daddy or Grandma make a quick run to the store for preemie onesies. If you're carrying multiples or are otherwise at especially high risk of delivering early, it couldn't hurt to have a preemie outfit or two on hand, just to be prepared. Don't stress too much about what baby will wear in those first few days anyway. They are so little at that point and don't do much other than sleep, that even just a few basic onesies or baby T-shirts will do the trick nicely.

month 5

> *I've found myself putting on tighter shirts just to see if my bump looks like a bump yet.* MrsC08

"Who's supposed to throw me a baby shower? And when should it be?"

There's no hard rule here: A shower can be hosted by whoever feels like honoring your baby-to-be. Often this is a close friend, a neighbor, a colleague, or yes—even an aunt, mom, or sister. Sometimes a group of friends and family will pitch in together to host your shower, splitting the costs, cooking, and other party prep. Traditionally, it was considered bad form for a family member to host, but that advice has become a little outdated. So if a family member offers to throw you a shindig, it's okay to accept. But, don't throw yourself a shower. As for your timing, months 6 through 8 are ideal. Before then, your bump may be MIA (a bigger belly makes for the cutest keepsake pics), and in month 9 you'll be getting uncomfortable. Plus, well, baby could pop out any minute. We know plenty of moms who tried cutting it close to their due date and wound up with a week-old baby in tow at their showers!

"Is it rude to register for gifts?"

Just the opposite: Shower guests aren't required to buy off your registry (or to buy you anything at all). The registry is simply a wish list—a convenience to help guide them to the goods you want and need . . . if they want the help. That said, you should never expect to receive only gifts you registered for, and you should never dis a friend who goes off the registry. It probably means they were putting extra thought and effort into the search for the perfect gift!

"When should I register?"

If you haven't started a registry already, go ahead and get it going. Your shower hosts will probably want to include your registry information on the invitations. Plus, it can take some time to scope out your ideal gear. (Use our checklist on page 81 to help you determine what you need and then log onto TheBump.com/registry to start your list.) Just be careful registering for clothes—if your shower isn't happening for a month or two, it's likely the items you choose will already be out of stock when folks start shopping.

"Is it okay to just ask for money as a baby shower gift?"

Sorry, but no. While we all have more uses for cash than 32 fleece blankets, you'd be out of line for requesting it. No one is obligated to give you (or baby) a gift, so what to give should be totally left up to the gift giver. Saving for something specific? Well, in that case, it's okay to throw that out as an option if—and only if—someone specifically asks what you need. ("We're kind of low on burp cloths, or you could just chip in toward the jogging stroller we're trying to buy" is much nicer than "We'd rather you just give us money.")

"We can't settle on the right name! Where can we find ideas?"

Besides flipping through name books and playing with online naming tools (time for a shameless plug: We have a fun one at TheBump.com!), try simply keeping your eyes and ears open as you go about your day. Read

green

Aside from being the first color that baby can see, green is calming. A soothing sight after a sleepless night or two.

orange

This trendy color for the nursery is warm and comforting. It's also equally appropriate for a girl's or boy's room.

"can I paint the nursery?"

Depends on what you mean here. It's okay for the nursery to be painted, but not a great idea for you to paint it. You could get hurt or put a serious knot in your back from all of the repetitive motion. Plus, even being around fresh paint is a no-no for pregnant women due to toxic fumes. Whoever paints should take some precautions. Today most manufacturers offer low-VOC or no-VOC options. (VOC stands for "volatile organic compounds.") These new paints emit little or no fumes, drastically reducing the health risks to you and baby. While they're a much better option than traditional paint, there's no guarantee even these are totally safe. So keep the windows open, and don't eat or drink near the work area. Take special caution if your house was built or decorated before 1978 when lead paint was banned. If you have the slightest suspicion that you have lead paint, leave the house while it's being removed. Inhaling the dust can be harmful to both you and baby.

purple

Cool colors like blue and purple often help to soothe babies. For a fun look in the nursery, pair light purple with its color-wheel opposite, green. Try the contrasting color on trim or accessories.

yellow

Bright yellow is energizing and can be kind of intense, so opt for a toned-down shade for baby's room.

nursery

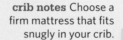

change up Convert any dresser into a changing table: Screw in a safety railing around the perimeter and add plush pad.

crib notes Choose a firm mattress that fits snugly in your crib.

trash talk A small pail with a lid is all you really need for diaper disposal. Just empty daily.

underfoot Spills and messes are inevitable: Choose durable flooring and add rugs.

the credits after the movies you watch, check out the captions under photos in the paper, and listen up when you're waiting in line at the store. (Just try not to be too creepy about it.) We know one mom-to-be that searched her company's international e-mail directory for inspiration and another that scoured the shelves at her local bookstore looking out for authors with interesting names. If you're stuck, brainstorming works well too. Sit down with your partner and jot down all the names that come to mind (favorite teacher, great-grandpa, the cute kid in that Lifetime movie . . . anything goes). Don't stress about it, baby doesn't really need a name until you leave the hospital. Plenty of parents make the final call on delivery day. Take your time and find a name that fits your new family to a T.

"We're keeping the name a secret until delivery, but people keep asking. How can we get them to back off?"

Have you tried saying, "Back off!"? That's about as good as you can do, short of fibbing a bit. Phrases like, "We're still trying to decide," might save you more grief than, "We're not telling," which begs for a follow-up question about why. If you've already made it clear that you're keeping names under wraps and get the inevitable, "Come on, you can just tell me," explain how much you're looking forward to introducing the baby in a few months—and then change the subject pronto. If you're firm about your decision and don't seem likely to give in, they'll be quicker to take the hint and drop it.

"When is a good time to start putting together my nursery?"

Most of our pregnant pals say they're aiming for the second trimester. After all, this is the time in pregnancy when you'll feel most up to it, and decorating plans may become more clear if you're peeking at baby's sex. So get to work! Even if you aren't quite ready to start painting, it's best to go ahead and pick out the major furniture in the next month or so—it can take several weeks to arrive and most likely more than one to trip to the store to pick it out. Make sure to measure your nursery before you head out to shop, and bring a tape measure with you to the store so that you make sure the things you pick out will fit into your baby room.

month 5

"How can I stay comfortable when I have to travel?"

Since you're generally feeling pretty good, the second trimester is great for traveling, as long as you take a couple of precautions. Here are a few tips to keep yourself (and baby!) safe and comfortable.

- Circulation is the key. Get up and walk around at least once an hour, and wiggle or massage your legs every few minutes while sitting. (Same goes for any time you're seated for an extended period of time while pregnant.) Keeping the blood flowing reduces the risk of developing throbbing varicose veins, thrombosis (blood clots), and swollen feet and ankles.
- Wear your seat belt across your thighs and tucked below your belly.

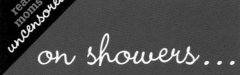

real moms uncensored

on showers...

In the last few years, most of the baby showers I've gone to have been coed, and at first the men were awkward, but throw in a few fun games and they LOVE it.
marinewifebarker

I threw my sister-in-law a mixed baby shower and everyone had a great time. It was nice to include the men, and her husband appreciated being able to invite HIS friends. *beansi*

I thought people would buy little things, like towels and sheets, but everyone bought clothes and blankets, which I am very thankful for! We'll have one stylish baby! *LarloBlue*

• Prop your feet up to help blood flow. If you're flying, try using a carry-on item stashed under the seat in front of you or put your feet up on an available seat.
• Avoid travel-induced dehydration by loading up on non-caffeinated fluids.
• To stay comfortable, request an aisle seat in the front half of the plane. This will give you a smoother ride and make it easier to get up and walk around.
• Try a back-support cushion or pillow. When traveling by car, push your seat back as far as possible to get more legroom. And, of course, make sure you stop for bathroom breaks periodically along the way.

"I'm dying for a little pampering. Are any spa treatments off-limits?"

Sounds like a treat . . . and one that you clearly deserve! As long as you're up front with the spa staff about your pregnancy, you should be fine with most treatments. Some spas actually offer packages for pregnant women that include specialized massages and intense foot rubs. Avoid heat treatments like saunas, hot tubs, tanning beds, and body wraps, because increased body temperature can harm baby. You may want to steer clear of facials (or look for a treatment that uses only natural products) if your skin is super-sensitive. Whatever treatment you choose, make sure the aesthetician is aware of your bump. And, as a rule of thumb, it's always a good idea to check with your OB to make sure that she's okay with the treatment that you're planning to get.

checklist

"what should I register for?"

Baby stores have huge lists of things to buy. Here's what you really need.

furniture/bedding

○ crib
○ crib mattress and covers
○ 2–3 fitted crib sheets
○ dresser

gear

○ high chair
○ swing
○ bouncer seat or rocker
○ car seat
○ car seat head support
○ car window shade
○ stroller
○ umbrella stroller
○ baby sling or carrier
○ diaper bag
○ changing mat
○ diaper pail and liner refills
○ activity mat

safety/health

○ baby monitor
○ pacifiers
○ thermometer
○ medicine dropper
○ nasal aspirator
○ baby nail clippers
○ first-aid kit
○ infant bathtub
○ 4–6 hooded bath towels
○ 6–8 washcloths
○ baby shampoo and wash
○ brush and comb set
○ diaper cream

layette/clothing

○ 4–6 undershirts
○ 4–6 receiving blankets
○ 4–6 long-sleeved onesies
○ 4–6 footed outfits
○ 4–6 sleep sacks
○ caps/mittens

feeding

○ 4–8 bibs
○ burp cloths
○ 10–16 bottles and nipples
○ disposable bottle liners
○ insulated bottle tote
○ bottle brush
○ bottle sterilizer
○ bottle warmer
○ dishwasher caddy
○ breast pump and accessories
○ breast milk storage containers or bags
○ 1–3 nursing bras
○ breast pads
○ nipple cream
○ nursing pillow

month 5

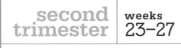

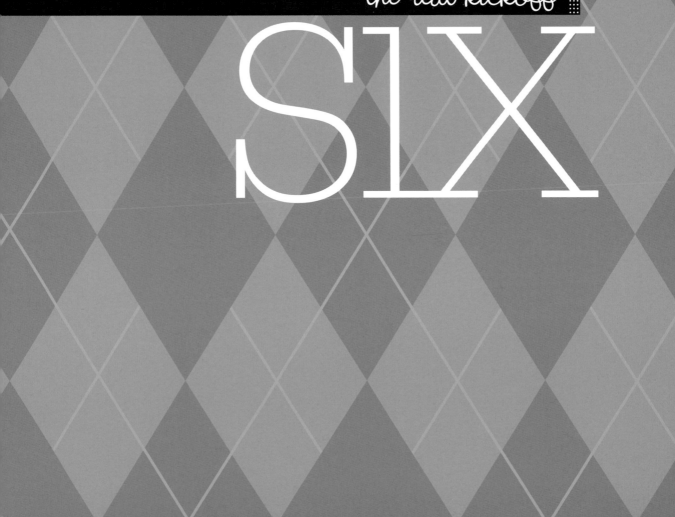

chapter 6

month

the real kickoff

SIX

still feeling good? Take it slow and enjoy these last weeks of the second trimester: Your bump's getting big, your baby's kicking up a storm, and you're still mobile enough to get around (pretty) easily. You might be feeling a little more in tune with baby now that his somersaults are consistent. Go ahead and have a chat with that adorable little alien growing inside you and play your favorite music—baby's ears are well developed by week 24. Now's also the time to start thinking seriously about your birth plan and figure out what you want (and don't want) to happen when you go into labor.

your to-do list

- Register for your shower gifts
- Schedule a glucose tolerance test
- Prepare a birth plan

Get the 411 on baby registries at TheBump.com/reg101

what you're in for . . .

" SHE'S KICKING LIKE CRAZY.

I have an outie now.

holy #!*?— hemorrhoids!

hmm . . . I don't remember that—what's it called again?

I DON'T CARE THAT I'M WEARING SNEAKERS WITH A SKIRT— I'M COMFORTABLE.

I have gas. A lot of it.

I'M SO HUNGRY.

INSANELY. ITCHY. BELLY. "

on your mind...

▌at the ob's office

"What's the glucose tolerance test like? What do the results mean?"

The glucose tolerance test (done sometime between weeks 24 and 28) is part of the screening for gestational diabetes. It goes something like this: You'll start fasting at midnight the night before the test. At your appointment, you'll chug a cup of incredibly sweet, syrupy liquid (it's called Glucola and contains 50 g glucose). You wait an hour. They take a sample of your blood to see how your body is reacting to the glucose. If the results are negative, you're done. If they're positive, you'll need to schedule another screening, called the 100-gram oral glucose

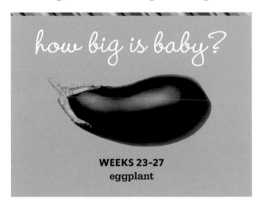

how big is baby?

WEEKS 23-27
eggplant

tolerance test, where they'll test you four times over a 3-hour time span. (Bring a book.) Lots of women fail the first test and pass the second with flying colors, but if two out of the four test results show abnormality, you'll be diagnosed with gestational diabetes and will need to talk with your OB about a health plan for the rest of your pregnancy.

"What's preeclampsia?"

Preeclampsia (also known as toxemia or pregnancy-induced hypertension) is diagnosed if, after week 20, you've got both high blood pressure and protein in your urine. The cause is a bit of a mystery, but the consequences are clear. With preeclampsia, blood vessels constrict and reduce blood flow, which can affect the liver, kidneys, and brain. The blood flow to baby also may be interrupted, which, in severe cases, can lead to poor growth, insufficient amniotic fluid, or the placenta peeling away from the uterus. Preeclampsia is fairly rare (5 to 10 percent of pregnancies). There seems to be a genetic link, so pay special attention to warning signs if your mom had it. Your risk goes up if you have chronic hypertension, blood clotting disorders, diabetes, kidney disease, or certain autoimmune diseases, or if you're overweight, older than 40 or younger than 20, or carrying multiples. Keep an eye on your body, and let your doctor know if your hands, face, or feet swell excessively or if you gain more than 4 pounds in one week. Some of the other warning signs include change in vision, intense pain in the upper abdomen, nausea, vomiting, and severe headaches. If you're diagnosed, your doctor will monitor you closely, limit your activities, and may induce labor a bit early.

Luckily, moms and babies dealing with preeclampsia usually turn out just fine if the disorder is detected early. Your best defense: Keep all of your prenatal appointments (your doctor screens for preeclampsia every time)

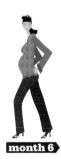

month 6

and watch for the warning signs. Also, some studies show that keeping weight down, taking vitamins, eating right, and minimizing stress can reduce your chances of getting preeclampsia. (One more reason to treat your body with extra TLC.)

"What are Braxton Hicks contractions? When do they start?"

Braxton Hicks contractions are relatively painless contractions of your uterus that begin as early as week 6 (though you don't feel them until around mid pregnancy, and some women don't notice them at all). Some mamas-to-be say it feels like your stomach is squeezing and getting hard or inflating like a balloon. Drinking water or taking a warm bath should relieve any discomfort. There's really nothing to worry about unless you're less than 37 weeks along and you feel more than four contractions an hour, which could be a sign of preterm labor.

"I've heard that 24 weeks = viability. What does this really mean?"

Generally, 24 weeks is the earliest that most OBs think your baby has a chance of surviving in the outside world. This means that if you were to go into preterm labor that couldn't be stopped—or if baby were otherwise in serious trouble and had to be delivered—after you've hit week 24, your baby would have a shot at making it. But, baby would definitely be in for a long stay in intensive care, and would be at high risk for serious problems down the road.

▌in your head

"What's a doula? Do I need one?"

A doula is a person (almost always a woman) who's been trained to help you make it through childbirth and then some. Though she doesn't have a medical background, she does (or should) have doula certification that enables her to offer physical and emotional support, and to advocate for you during labor and delivery. Experienced doulas know about positioning, soothing touch, relaxation techniques, and other tricks to keep you comfortable and help you progress through labor. Many (called postpartum doulas) will also help you out at home for the first days or weeks of baby's life, doing whatever is needed to help you adjust (like cooking, shopping, and helping you learn to care for baby). A doula can be a big asset, especially if you go the drug-free route. To find one near you, ask your OB for a recommendation or try the Doula Organization of North America's finder at DONA.org.

"Any tips for do-it-yourself maternity picture poses?"

Hey, you're the artist. Think about how you can use the photos to communicate how you've been feeling. Had a wacky dream? Use it as inspiration. Craving certain foods? Balance them on your belly. Just felt like your belly finally "popped," go in for a closeup. You can also use the camera to try and capture other stuff that's going on in your life during your pregnancy—try incorporating your pets, other children, and, of course, your partner.

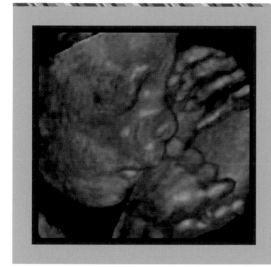

what baby's up to

- little ears develop
- face is fully formed—minus the baby fat
- skin is becoming more opaque
- baby's learning to distinguish right side up from upside down
- eyes are forming—soon she'll be trying out her blinking skills

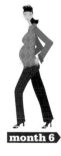

month 6

"I think I'd like to change my work schedule after baby. Should I talk to my boss about it now? How?"

If you're hoping to switch things up once your maternity leave is over, it is probably best to lay your ideas on the table now. First, make sure you're clear on what your company's policies state (like whether part of your leave would be covered by disability insurance, and whether you'd retain health insurance with your new schedule). Once you've done your homework, write up a detailed proposal for your boss. Go ahead and flesh out exactly how your ideal schedule would work. Are you thinking part-time? Flex time? Do you want to telecommute? As well as what sort of workload you could handle in that amount of time. It may also help to mention who could take on any responsibilities you'll be casting aside, and how you'll train them.

Next, set up a meeting and have a heart to heart with the boss. She'll appreciate that you've organized the details in a way that makes the plan easy to implement, upping your chances of getting your way. Talk it out (be ready to compromise) and make a plan. Be sure to get the final agreement in writing (and send a copy to your human resources department) to avoid misunderstandings later on. (Disclaimer: Only you know your boss and your company. We can't promise that she'll go for it.)

"Do I really need a birth plan?"

A "birth plan" is really just a way for you to communicate with your partner, doctors, and nurses about delivery-day issues like pain meds, people involved, episiotomies, and cord cutting. The plan can be anything from a simple, "I want to avoid interventions if at all possible," or, "I'd like you to do whatever you can to keep me from feeling pain," to a full page of desires for labor and childbirth.

If you write up a plan, it's important to talk everything over with your OB to be certain it's realistic and falls in line with hospital policies. After you've cleared your plan with your doctor, make sure there's a copy in your chart and a few copies in the bag you'll take to the hospital. (Have your labor partner hand them out to the labor nurses when you arrive.) If a birth plan is in place, everyone involved in delivery can be reminded of your wishes if decisions need to be made. That way, you can just focus on the pushing!

It's fine to go without a birth plan too. Just make sure your labor coach is up to speed on how you feel about different options, since you may not feel much like thinking through big decisions between contractions. And if you do make a written plan, remember that it's nothing but a wish list of basic guidelines. Your (and baby's!) health and safety come first, and birth plans often change.

> I plan to write a simple, flexible birth plan with the understanding that things may have to change. Why not have something written down so you don't have to think when you're in the moment?
>
> *qmommy*

⬛ is it normal?

"I'm swelling—I know this is normal, but when should I worry?"

You're right that it's normal—nearly all women swell up at least a little, particularly their feet and ankles. Annoying? Yes. Dangerous? Not usually. Call your doctor if your face swells, if your hands puff up more than just a little, or if your ankles or feet swell very suddenly. This can be a sign of preeclampsia. Also call if one leg is much more swollen than the other, which can sometimes signal a blood clot.

"Ack! Cankles! Is there any kind of cure?"

More than one mama has seen her calves and ankles merge into one. For everyday swelling, R&R is your best bet. Get off your feet and lie down (preferably on your left side) whenever possible. When you sit, elevate your feet, don't cross your ankles or legs, and stretch frequently. Also, get up and walk around to keep your blood moving. Drink plenty of water (we know it sounds counterintuitive, but it works). Pregnancy support hose can also bring sweet relief—they're designed to squeeze your legs in a way that prevents water retention, and they'll help out with varicose and spider veins too. Finally, take some comfort in the fact that your lovely, slim ankles will reappear one day.

"I have terrible gas! What's going on . . . and what can I do?"

At least the gas is for a good cause: The hormone progesterone is relaxing smooth muscles in your gastrointestinal tract to make your gut work slower, giving your body

"what's included in a birth plan?"

Use this short version of our easy, fill-in-the-blank birth plan to prepare yourself for delivery and communicate what you want to your medical team.

my delivery is planned as:
- Vaginal
- C-section
- Water birth
- Vaginal Birth After Cesarean

I'd like . . .
- Partner
- Parents
- Doula
- Other

. . . present before and/or during labor

for pain relief, I'd like to use:
- Acupressure
- Acupuncture
- Breathing techniques
- Cold therapy and/or hot therapy
- Demerol
- Hypnosis
- Massage
- Meditation
- Reflexology
- Standard epidural
- Transcutaneous Elictrical Nerve Stimulator
- Walking epidural
- Nothing

during labor I'd like . . .
- Music played (which I'll provide)
- The lights dimmed
- The room as quiet as possible
- As few interruptions as possible
- As few vaginal exams as possible
- Hospital staff limited to my own doctor and nurses
- To wear my own clothes
- To wear my contact lenses
- My partner to film and/or take pictures
- My partner to be present
- To stay hydrated with clear liquids and ice chips
- To eat and drink as approved

as my baby is delivered, I'd like to:
- Push spontaneously
- Push as directed
- Push with no time limits, as long as the baby and I aren't at risk
- Use a mirror to see baby crown
- Touch the head as it crowns
- Avoid forceps usage
- Avoid vacuum extraction
- Use whatever methods my doctor deems necessary

month 6

more time to snatch up nutrients from your food and take them to baby. Unfortunately, a slower gut can translate into some serious belches and toots. Soon your growing uterus will start pushing up on your stomach and down on your rectum, too, compounding the problem. To help relieve the pressure, eat small, regular meals and stay away from foods that tend to give you gas. You know the culprits: fried stuff, dairy, beans, dried fruit, Brussels sprouts, cabbage, and so on. Eating and drinking slowly will also keep you from swallowing excess air. Taking a yoga class can help settle things down too. And, ward off constipation (a big gas-inducer) with plenty of liquids and high-fiber foods.

"I'm on my feet a ton at work. What can I do to ease the foot and back pain?"

Between your shifting center of balance, all that extra weight, and loosening ligaments, it's no wonder that you're aching. If you can't get off your feet (ask for breaks and prop up your tootsies when you can!), be sure to wear comfy shoes with good support, and try adding a gel insole—they make them for heels now too! Speaking of heels, they aren't a total no-no. Retire your stilettos, but keep out the kitten heels—1½- to 2-inch heels may actually provide extra support for your back. If you start to have a lot of trouble with swelling, consider support hose, which can keep the blood from pooling in your feet. You

might also benefit from a pregnancy support belt, especially as you grow even larger. It can seriously ease the stress on your back. (Bonus: Some moms say it takes a load off their bladder too!) Also, make a special effort to maintain good posture—your back (make that your whole body) will thank you.

"I just realized I have hemorrhoids! What can I do about them?"

You've got extra blood flowing through your veins right now, and it can sometimes pool up in the parts of your body most affected by gravity (such as, yes, the rectum). The result is swollen, itchy varicose veins, and when these come where the sun don't shine, they're called hemorrhoids. Your growing uterus is also adding pressure to the region, making it prone to swelling. Talk to your OB about creams and suppositories that you can use to ease the pain, experiment with hot or cold packs, or try witch hazel pads and sitz baths (soaking the area in a little hot water). Constipation (and the straining it leads to) may also be the culprit, so make an extra effort stay hydrated and eat lots of fiber. If you still can't get regular, ask your doctor which stool softeners are safe. Excess weight can make hemorrhoids worse, so try to stay within your doctor's recommended guidelines, and don't forget to exercise—even if it's not so comfortable right now. When you get moving, you'll ease

> I thought I was going to get away with no hemorrhoids this time, but wrong! I used the Preparation H wipes and ointment. It wasn't a big deal and went away pretty fast.
> amber*n*scott

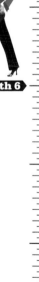

month 6

the pressure on the veins in your pelvic area. (It'll help the constipation too.) And finally, keep up your Kegels—they can help increase circulation to the area.

"I don't think I've felt the baby kick in awhile and it's worrying me. How can I make her kick?"

You can help nudge baby into wiggling with a glass of cold milk (or anything else chilly and sweet) and lying on your side to increase blood flow to her. Or try one of our favorite pastimes: The remote control trick. Drink something sweet, then lie back in a recliner (or on the couch propped up with pillows) with the TV remote balanced on your belly. You'll see it move when baby bounces!

If you still don't feel any kicks, or don't get ten kicks in an hour when you do your counts, get in touch with your OB.

"I'm waking up with awful leg cramps! How can I keep from getting them?"

Leg cramps are common as you enter the last months of pregnancy. Doctors aren't sure why, but they suspect it has something to do with changes in circulation, the extra weight you're carrying, or baby pressing on nerves and blood vessels. Whatever the reason, they can be a serious pain.

To keep cramps at bay, try stretching and massaging your calves before bed and in the morning, and adding bananas to your diet (some experts think the potassium might help). If you find yourself stretching out your legs when you lie in bed, don't point your

real moms uncensored

on travel...

Originally, I was allowed to fly until 22 weeks, but my OB won't let me now, so no more vacations for me.
femmefatalenat01

I always made sure to get an aisle seat since I had to pee so much!
tarzanswife

I flew three times when I was pregnant. Once I took my shoes off during the flight, and when I tried to put them back on at the end, my feet were too swollen!
sunny1in tucson

We went to Florida when I was about 22 weeks and I was already pretty big, so the flight was uncomfortable. I'd say 20 weeks is the latest I would travel.
home_slice

toes! (Chances are, they get stuck there.) When the cramps come on, enlist your partner to grab your leg and flex your feet, or stand and do a lunge beside the bed. Once it eases up a little, walking around for a few minutes can help relax the muscle.

"I just found the car keys in the fridge. Is this baby making me lose my mind?"

There aren't scientific studies to prove it, but we (and nearly all of our mom friends) have been there too. The best guesses are that hormones, lack of sleep, and distracted minds are to blame. Try to keep it together by making lots of lists, eating a well-balanced diet, snacking often, taking your prenatal vitamins, and getting as much rest as you can. And don't worry—it isn't permanent. One study actually suggested that mothers wind up sharper in the long run, so there's plenty of sanity to look forward to!

"My boobs are totally killing me! Why and when will it end?"

Breast tenderness is one of the first signs of pregnancy, and while it usually fades by the end of the first trimester, it can last longer for some women. We've heard of moms-to-be well into their second trimester describe the feeling "like someone put jumper cables on my nipples every time a cool breeze goes by." Your best defense: a good supportive bra (some women even like to wear a pregnancy sleep bra at night) along with liberal amounts of a heavy balm to prevent chafing. See more on bras on page 38.

is it safe to . . .

"When do I have to stop flying?"

Good news: You're still clear for a couple more weeks—doctors say it's fine for you to travel until as late as week 36 as long as you're having a healthy pregnancy. When you're airborne, drink lots of water and get up to take a walk down the aisle every hour or two to get your blood flowing and reduce the risk of blood clots. You may want to stay grounded earlier if you're carrying multiples, though. Talk to your doctor for specific recommendations.

"What can baby hear? Do I need to stay away from loud noise?"

Those tiny inner ears have been forming since month 4, but now they're becoming well developed. Go ahead and sing, chat, read, and play your favorite tunes for your mini-me. Studies show that, while lots of sounds are filtered out by the uterine wall and amniotic fluid, baby is able to hear, respond to, and remember sounds from his time in the womb. It's the lower-frequency noises that make it through, so go heavy on the bass. As for volume, you should be fine taking in a concert or sitting by a horde of screaming football fans—just be ready for baby to react to all the hoopla, especially during the last trimester. The jury's still out on whether frequent loud noises are truly safe. If you work in an especially noisy place (we're talking about loud machinery here; not your annoying cube-mates), talk with your OB about making a new plan.

"I'm sick of walking. What are some fun ways to get my exercise in while I'm pregnant?"

Thirty minutes of exercise a day (with your OB's approval), can lower your risk of complications like diabetes and preeclampsia. Plus, it's associated with shorter labors and quicker recoveries—pretty good incentives if you ask us. No matter what new exercise you try, make sure to tell the instructor you're pregnant so she can modify moves as necessary.

month 6

swimming
WHY IT'S GOOD The pool lets you feel weightless for a change, taking a load off joints and compressed organs while you work a wide range of muscle groups.
WHAT TO TRY Gentle laps or a basic water aerobics class

yoga
WHY IT'S GOOD Not only is yoga great for your body, you'll learn breathing and relaxation techniques that can be a big help during labor, and positions to try if you'll be going sans epidural.
WHAT TO TRY Prenatal yoga or a basic, level-one class

pilates
WHY IT'S GOOD Since it focuses on your core, Pilates can improve your posture, prevent backaches, and even help when it's time for you to push.
WHAT TO TRY Prenatal mat classes, or a basic mat class

belly dancing
WHY IT'S GOOD The traditional Middle Eastern dance was used in ancient times to help women get ready for childbirth, soothing baby and preparing the body for the delivery.
WHAT TO TRY Any class you can find! Or a good DVD

▌the day-to-day

"When do we need to start figuring out what to do about child care?"

Last week. Just kidding (sort of)—the answer to this one depends on where you live and what kind of care you're looking for. If you're shooting for a day care facility (stimulating environment, interaction with other kids), you'll probably need to apply pronto. Day cares in major cities can have waiting lists out the wazoo (as in 9 to 12 months or more). Prefer an in-home nanny (personal attention; more flexible schedules; higher cost)? Put your feelers out for recommendations, but you should be okay holding off on interviews until baby's around to help pick his match.

"Should I be doing kick counts?"

Kick counts are an easy way to check in on baby and catch problems before they get out of hand. There are lots of different ways to count baby's karate chops, so ask your OB for specific suggestions. A common way is to time how long it takes to feel ten movements. Pick a time every day to tune into your tummy and simply count the kicks, swishes, bumps, and jabs. If you tally ten movements in under an hour, check it off your list until tomorrow. If it takes longer than two hours, or if you notice any big deviations from the norm (like, if it usually take 15 minutes, but starts taking 55 minutes), play it safe and give your OB a ring.

Start kick counts as soon as you've hit a point in pregnancy where you feel baby squirming on a regular basis, and do your counts at a time of day when baby's usually most active, like after dinner or when you lie down in bed at night. If things seem slow, try downing a glass of cold milk—the sugar and temperature can hype baby up—and lying on your left side, which increases blood flow.

"What are Kegels? How do I do them?"

Kegels are exercises that help strengthen the muscles on your pelvic floor, which support your uterus, bladder, and bowel. What's the point? Do these, and you'll be less likely to pee your pants when baby begins pressing on your bladder in the third trimester. They'll help with similar problems post-delivery, too. Plus, one 2004 study even showed that Kegels can shorten the second phase of labor (the pushing part). Add in the fact that Kegels are known to help out in the bedroom (they make it easier to orgasm), and this is one exercise you don't want to slack on.

There are different ways to do a Kegel, and some experts think it's best to mix it up. First, find the right muscles by attempting to stop your urine mid-stream a couple of times. Feel the muscles that you use? Those are the Kegels. (Don't routinely practice your Kegels while you tinkle, though. It can actually weaken the muscles.) Now imagine smoothly drawing those pelvic floor muscles up like an elevator. Hold at the top for a count of 10; then slowly lower muscles to the starting position. Repeat ten times. For some variation, quickly contract and release the muscles ten times in a row. Take a break, and then repeat the exercise ten more times.

chart

kick-count tracker

Keep a record of baby's every move throughout your pregnancy.

I am in the _____ week of my pregnancy.

	mon	tues	wed	thurs	fri	sat	sun
	___	___	___	___	___	___	___
start time	:	:	:	:	:	:	:
stop time	:	:	:	:	:	:	:
minutes to reach 10							

I am in the _____ week of my pregnancy.

	mon	tues	wed	thurs	fri	sat	sun
	___	___	___	___	___	___	___
start time	:	:	:	:	:	:	:
stop time	:	:	:	:	:	:	:
minutes to reach 10							

I am in the _____ week of my pregnancy.

	mon	tues	wed	thurs	fri	sat	sun
	___	___	___	___	___	___	___
start time	:	:	:	:	:	:	:
stop time	:	:	:	:	:	:	:
minutes to reach 10							

I am in the _____ week of my pregnancy.

	mon	tues	wed	thurs	fri	sat	sun
	___	___	___	___	___	___	___
start time	:	:	:	:	:	:	:
stop time	:	:	:	:	:	:	:
minutes to reach 10							

month 6

"how do I choose a stroller?"

Buying a stroller can be almost as confusing as buying a car. A newborn needs a seat that either fully reclines or accommodates an infant carrier. If you go for the carrier, make sure it's easy to lock into the stroller. After infancy, things get a little more complicated. Use this flowchart to figure out what fits best with your lifestyle.

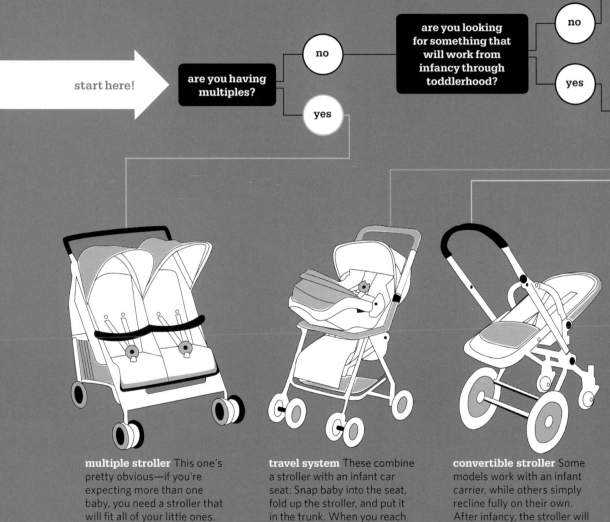

start here! → **are you having multiples?**

no → **are you looking for something that will work from infancy through toddlerhood?**

no

yes

yes

multiple stroller This one's pretty obvious—if you're expecting more than one baby, you need a stroller that will fit all of your little ones.

travel system These combine a stroller with an infant car seat: Snap baby into the seat, fold up the stroller, and put it in the trunk. When you reach your destination, unlatch the seat from the car and place it (and baby) into the stroller.

convertible stroller Some models work with an infant carrier, while others simply recline fully on their own. After infancy, the stroller will continue to work with a stroller seat attachment until baby hits toddlerhood.

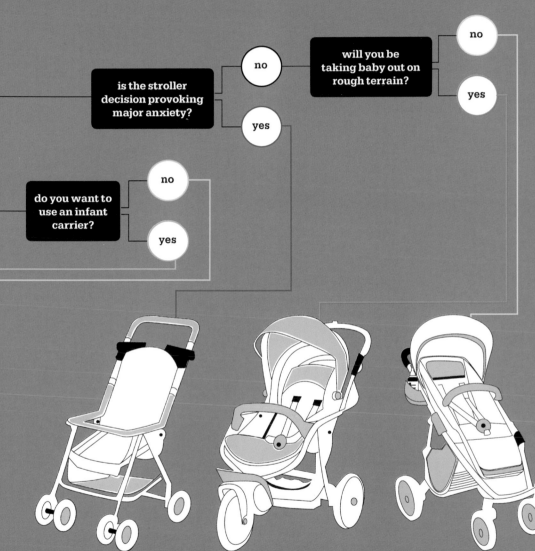

is the stroller decision provoking major anxiety?

no

will you be taking baby out on rough terrain?

no

yes

yes

do you want to use an infant carrier?

no

yes

month 6

stroller frame Similar to the travel system, you just snap baby's car seat right into the frame. When baby outgrows the car seat, you'll have to get an actual stroller.

all-terrain/jogging stroller Designed for hikes, runs, and uneven surfaces, these durable strollers can be hard to manage on stairs and elevators. Keep in mind, most aren't appropriate for babies younger than six months.

umbrella stroller Relatively inexpensive and easy to maneuver and fold, these are a convenient option for babies who can sit up on their own. (Like all-terrain strollers, you'll need to use something else until baby reaches that point.)

chapter 7

month

officially huge

seven

you've made it to the third trimester! The end is in sight, and you're probably still feeling semi-good—though some fatigue may be sneaking back in, you're running to the bathroom again, and it's getting tougher to tie your shoes. This is a good time to start making serious plans for your new life with a baby (finding a pediatrician, stocking up on bottles, familiarizing yourself with the carseat, trying not to freak out). You're probably starting to think about the reality of labor and delivery, too. Yes, this baby is going to eventually come out. And if you think your belly is ginormous now, just wait—it's still got a long way to go!

your to-do list

- **Find a pediatrician**
- **Take a tour of the maternity ward**
- **Preregister with the hospital**
- **Sign up for a breastfeeding class**

Get our complete pediatrician checklist at TheBump.com/pedi

what you're in for...

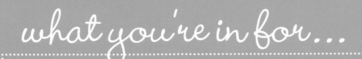

66 **time's flying.**

ouch! **my boobs just started leaking.**

WHAT DOES IT MEAN IF I MEASURE BIG?

I have to pee all the time.

I'm such a klutz.

I'm still feeling so tired.

MY FEET ARE EVEN MORE SWOLLEN!

insanely itchy belly and boobs! 99

on your mind...

▌at the ob's office

"What does it mean if I'm measuring too small or too big at the doctor's office?"

In general, after 20 weeks, your fundal height (the distance from your pubic bone to the top of your uterus) should pretty much equal the number of weeks you've been pregnant. So, if you start measuring more than two centimeters off in either direction, your OB will probably schedule you for an ultrasound to check things out.

POSSIBLE REASONS FOR MEASURING LARGE

- You simply have a big, healthy baby
- Your due date was wrong
- You're carrying twins or more
- You have too much amniotic fluid

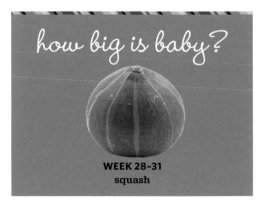

how big is baby?

WEEK 28–31
squash

- Baby is especially high in the uterus
- You have gestational diabetes (which can lead to bigger babies)

POSSIBLE REASONS FOR MEASURING SMALL

- You have a small baby
- Your due date was wrong
- There could be an intrauterine growth restriction which is when baby is below the tenth percentile for its age; it could be due to many reasons: placenta problems, heart disease in the mother, even high altitudes
- You have too little amniotic fluid

"Will my baby come early? How can I prevent that from happening?"

Preterm birth (delivery before week 37) affects around 12 percent of pregnancies in the US. The risk is higher if you have an incompetent cervix (sounds harsh, but just means it opens prematurely), have vaginal bleeding in the second or third trimester, went into preterm labor in a prior pregnancy, or if you're carrying multiples, are a smoker, underweight, under 20, or over 35.

You can't always prevent preterm labor, but you can use these tips to lower your risk:

- Start prenatal care asap, and keep all of your OB appointments
- Maintain a healthy pregnancy weight
- Drink lots of water
- Don't smoke or use drugs
- Call your doctor anytime you feel sick
- Don't stress

To protect yourself and baby, get familiar with preterm labor symptoms. If you see them coming and get to the doctor quickly, baby might be convinced to stay put. Keep on the lookout for contractions that occur four or more times in an hour, lower back pain, pelvic pressure, vaginal discharge tinged with blood, menstrual-like cramping, or diarrhea. And never, ever feel shy about calling your doctor if you're worried.

month 7

in your head

"I just realized that this baby actually has to come OUT. I'm starting to panic!"
First, know that it's completely normal to be nervous. If you start feeling overwhelmed, it might help to think of all the women throughout history who gave birth before you (and how many didn't enjoy the luxury of a hospital room and an OB!). Every single person in the world was born, and most of them came out of vaginas. That means there is a darn good chance you'll get through this just fine. If that rationale doesn't calm you, try finding something that does, like yoga, meditation, talking it out with a trusted friend, or reading about other moms' experiences.

"Can't I just schedule a c-section and avoid the whole pushing-out-the-baby ordeal?"
Maybe. We know some doctors who say that elective cesarean sections are just fine, or even that they save a woman's pelvic floor from stresses that could lead to incontinence (aka peeing your pants) later in life. But we know plenty of others who think it's a bad idea to go under the knife without necessity. A c-section, after all, is major surgery and isn't without risks. You should also be aware that your health insurance might not cover an elective cesarean—look over your policy to be sure. If you do choose to schedule a c-section, try to cut it (no pun intended) as close as possible to 39 weeks. A recent study showed that baby is more likely to have health problems if he's delivered by c-section before 39 weeks or after 40 weeks.

> Aside from something being wrong with baby, I'm afraid of progressing really slowly and having a longer than average labor and farting—don't ask me why that freaks me out but it does. *12bailey18*

"If I fall, will it hurt the baby?"
The combo of a shifting center of balance and ligament-loosening hormones swimming around can definitely make you clumsy. First off, you can prevent falls by wearing comfortable shoes with non-skid soles (this is NOT the time for four-inch heels), holding onto railings on the stairs, avoiding slick surfaces, and being extra-careful in general. If you do happen to suffer a fall, don't panic. Baby is very well padded in her fluid-filled home, and isn't likely to be hurt at all. Do call your OB, though—she might want to check out baby's heartbeat, just to make sure all is well.

"Be honest—what exactly will a vaginal birth do to my vagina?"
Yes, pushing a human being out of such a small opening is scary to every one of us. Don't freak, though. Your body is amazing, and it's made to go through this. Here's the real-life scoop on what your vagina is in for. (If you don't want to know, don't read on.)

Will your vagina be exactly the same as it was before? No—probably not. Most couples report some degree of noticeable change . . . but they also tend to say it isn't so bad. Your vagina will do some serious stretching as

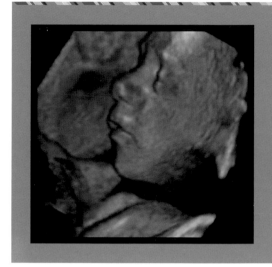

what baby's up to

- kicking extra hard and often
- packing on the fat layer
- brain is growing a bunch
- lungs begin to function
- lanugo starts to disappear
- has eyebrows and eyelashes
- has smooth, pink skin
- eyes have color (they might change after delivery)

baby slides out, and you will be swollen and bruised for a while. As you recover during the next couple of weeks, your vagina will gradually shrink back down (though maybe not all the way). To help regain muscle tone and tighten things up, keep up your Kegels, especially in the weeks following delivery. These exercises will also help to keep you from leaking urine after you deliver as well as after menopause (pretty common after the stresses of childbirth).

Your vagina may tear during delivery, or you might have an episiotomy (the doctor could make a cut to enlarge the opening). In either case, you'll likely be stitched up and will heal in 6 weeks or so. Your perineum (the skin between your vagina and rectum) could look noticeably different, depending on the degree of tearing and the skill of the person who did the stitching. If there's a

difference, don't worry, no one is really looking. You may also be left with a bit of scar tissue, which can be uncomfortable during your first attempts at postpartum sex. Each woman's experience is different, but you should feel back to normal (or close to it, at least) after a few (or a few dozen) rolls in the hay. One more temporary vagina alteration: You'll probably be really dry, especially if you're breastfeeding. Lube is your friend.

is it normal?

"Ahh! I have to pee all the time again. How can I cut down on bathroom trips?"
Between the masses of extra blood in your body (meaning more fluids running through your kidneys) and the pressure created by

month 7

your ever-expanding (shall we say giant?) uterus, it's no wonder you're always in the loo. You won't find complete relief until baby arrives, but here are three tips for spending a little less time on the toilet.

GET IT ALL OUT Make an effort to empty your bladder completely every time you pee. Lean forward to add a little bit of pressure to your bladder and get all the urine out. Bonus: This also helps prevent UTIs.

DRINK THE RIGHT STUFF Stay away from coffee, tea, and alcohol, all of which can keep you running to the ladies' room. (You should be steering clear of alcohol and more than two servings of caffeine daily anyway, of course.)

EASE UP IN THE EVENING Curbing your liquids in the hours before bedtime might make your nightly bathroom runs less frequent. If you go this route, just be sure to get plenty of fluids in the daytime—hydration is extra important as you move toward the big day.

is it safe?

"Can I give birth at home?"

Technically, you can give birth anywhere you want. Living rooms aren't exactly the most popular option for American moms (roughly 99 percent of births take place in a hospital), but stories of home births are popping up all over the media these days. Celebs like Cindy Crawford, Demi Moore, and Meryl Streep have chosen to skip the hospital for their deliveries. Proponents say home births

protect a woman from unnecessary drugs and episiotomies and that remaining in a comfortable, relaxed environment helps the birth to go smoothly. But, there's one pretty huge caveat: no emergency medical care. If you are considering a home birth, be sure to sit down and discuss all the pros, cons, and "what ifs" with your OB or midwife.

delivery countdown

"How do I preregister with the hospital? (And why do I have to?)"

Preregistering will take care of your basic admission paperwork, so your file is all ready to go on delivery day. If your hospital offers preregistration, it can save you some hassle—and maybe even get you into a room faster—when baby finally decides to make an appearance. Check with your hospital to find out what you need to do. Often, it's as simple as filling out a single form, and you may be able to do it over the telephone or online. It usually takes only a few minutes, and can save you or your partner from digging for your insurance card—and having to think—once you're in active labor.

"Are there exercises I can do that will make giving birth easier?"

Giving birth probably won't be "easy" no matter what you do, but it certainly does involve muscles, breathing, and endurance. Flexibility helps too—and all of these are

"I can't sleep! help!"

Between hormonal changes, a growing belly, a sore back, and a squished bladder, it's no wonder you're watching infomercials at 3 A.M. To help catch some (much needed!) zzzs, use these tips to wind down and get comfy.

- Reduce your fluid intake after 7 P.M. (to cut down on bathroom runs).
- Read a book (not about pregnancy) to get your mind off your anxieties.
- Drink a small cup of chamomile tea before bed (known for its relaxing benefits).
- Stay active. Low impact exercise can improve sleep.
- Ask your partner for a massage.
- Experiment with wedging pillows around your body to ease hip, back, or other pains.
- Take a warm bath.

things you can work on to help your body prepare for the hard work of labor. Here are a few exercises to try (just be sure to get the all-clear from your OB first).

HIP OPENERS Sit on the floor with the soles of your feet pressed together and your knees open wide in a diamond shape. Use your elbows to open the hips further, and hold for 30 to 60 seconds. Opening your hips helps to make room for baby's arrival.

AB CLENCHES You'll definitely need your abs when it's time to start pushing. (Yes, they might be stretched out, but they're still there.) Traditional crunches aren't practical though—you shouldn't lie on your back, and improper form could cause your abs to tear. Instead, sit or stand up straight and focus on pulling your navel back towards your spine. Hold it there for a few breaths, and release. Like Kegels, you can do these just about anywhere. Try to hold this pose as often as possible to protect and condition your abs.

MODERATE CARDIO Stay active by walking, swimming, or taking a prenatal workout class. You'll appreciate the lung capacity and heart conditioning when it comes time to breath through contractions.

"I overheard someone at the OB talking about a VBAC. What is that?"

It stands for "vaginal birth after cesarean." Not long ago, one c-section meant you were destined to have cesareans for every child, but now 60 to 80 percent of women who've had a c-section can give birth to future children the old-fashioned way. If you had a c-section for one child, bring up the idea of VBAC with your OB. Chances are that you'll be able to deliver vaginally this time around.

"I'm pregnant with twins. How early should I expect to go into labor?"

Twins tend to arrive sooner than singleton babies. While single babies develop for an average of 39 weeks, twins tend to appear around 35 weeks. (Triplets often arrive even sooner, by about 32 weeks; and quadruplets cook for an average of about 29 weeks.)

"If I am having twins, will I definitely need to have a c-section?"

Not necessarily. It depends on your babies' size and position. If they are both head-down, then you can deliver vaginally, and many twin moms do. No matter what, you'll need to deliver in a hospital, and you should find an OB skilled in twin deliveries to help ensure all goes well. (More babies mean a higher risk of complications.)

When you arrive at the hospital, you'll probably have an ultrasound to confirm that your babies are head-down and ready to go. Then, you'll labor just like a singleton mom. When it's time for delivery, you'll probably be wheeled into an operating room instead of a regular delivery room. This is in case one or both twins wind up needing an emergency c-section. (Sometimes the first twin can be born vaginally but the second one has to come by cesarean.) After your first twin arrives, your OB will check on your second to see if he's well positioned for delivery. If so, the

checklist

"what questions should I ask when I tour the maternity ward?"

Some Qs like "What will the room look like?" and "Where should we park?" will for sure be answered without asking, but you should come armed with anything (and everything) else you've been wondering. Here are some questions to get you started.

- Can I pre-register a couple of weeks before delivery? Can I do it online? (Getting some legal hoopla out of the way can be very freeing.)
- When we arrive, do we need to check in at the front desk first, or can I waddle straight to the maternity ward?
- What are the policies on cameras and video cameras?
- Are cell phones allowed?
- How many people are allowed in the delivery room?
- Can my partner stay the night?

- How soon after giving birth can I try to breastfeed?
- What are my chances for getting a private room? Will my insurance cover it?
- Will baby be able to stay in my room the whole time?
- Can the nursery staff look after baby if I need a break? How does that process work?
- What sort of breastfeeding support is offered? How does it work?
- Where and when are my other children allowed to be with me?

month 7

car seat

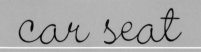

head support Look for a special insert to support infant's wobbly head. Only use one that comes with the seat.

harness A five-point harness is a must. Look for straps that are easy to adjust and a buckle that's not tricky to unlatch.

energy-absorbing foam During an accident, this is what keeps baby safe and protected from impact.

side protection Deep side walls and adequate barriers around the head protect baby from a side-impact accident.

comfort Does the material and padding feel soft and snuggly? This may sound like a luxury, but trust us —anything that helps soothe baby is essential those first few months.

registration Register your car seat so you'll be notified of any recalls or updates.

expiration date Yes, car seats have them. Normal lifespan is about 6 years.

blankets Jackets can affect the way baby sits in the car seat and impact how it performs, so it's better to dress baby normally, then keep him warm with blankets.

you'll also see

MIRRORS AND TOYS Though these may seem like great ways to keep baby distracted and calm during a car ride, they've got the potential of turning into hazardous flying objects during a car accident. Even seemingly innocuous toys that clip onto the car seat can be a problem, as they may affect the way it performs.

OB may break your water to encourage baby number two to move along. The contractions will restart soon (or you'll get some Pitocin to help them along), and you can then start pushing, the same way as before.

the day-to-day
"How do I find a pediatrician?"

Rule #1: Ask around. Good, old-fashioned word of mouth is the best way to find a great doctor. Ask friends and family members with kids, and you're sure to hear about a pedi or two that they just love. Can't think of who to ask? You can also corner new moms (in a nice way) for advice as they're picking up their tots from the nursery at church or shopping at a local baby store. They've been in your shoes, so chances are good they'll be happy to help. (Your pregnant belly will keep you from looking too creepy.) Online reviews can be helpful as well, as can moms on your local online message boards.

Log on to your insurance company's Web site (or give them a call) to access a list of local doctors who are covered by your plan. Once you've narrowed it down to a couple of candidates, begin making phone calls and setting up consultations (don't worry, these are usually free). A quick round of interviews will help you to find a great match. And remember not to stress too much: You can switch doctors at any time. This decision isn't permanent.

breastfeeding 411
"What are the benefits of breastfeeding?"

There's no doubt breast milk is the ideal food for baby. It contains the perfect mix of enzymes and antibodies, making breastfed babies less likely to have ear infections, colds, diarrhea, respiratory problems, allergies, and stomach bugs. Plus, nursing decreases future risk of obesity, diabetes, inflammatory bowel disease, childhood leukemia, and other forms of cancer. The list goes on and on. It's even been linked to higher IQs.

There are perks for you too. For one, it won't cost you a penny. Plus, it requires no preparation, is always wherever you are, and it comes out at the perfect temperature. The other bonus: It can help you drop your pregnancy pounds faster, help you heal more quickly down below, and has been linked to decreased breast cancer, uterine cancer, and osteoporosis rates.

"Do I need to do anything to prepare for breastfeeding?"

Breastfeeding can be tougher than it sounds, especially if you don't know what to expect. The best prep is to get educated: Take a breastfeeding class while you're pregnant, read up on the subject wherever you can, and chat with any breastfeeding friends. There are tons of Web sites and blogs that focus on breastfeeding, too. Every baby is different, but if you know the basics, you'll be more confident when baby actually has a go at your nipples. It's a good idea to seek

month 7

out resources for breastfeeding questions or help down the line. (Your OB or hospital can probably point you to a local lactation specialist.) As for any physical prep, like "toughening up" your nipples . . . nah, that's not really necessary.

"Will I have a harder time breastfeeding if I have small boobs?"

The amount of milk you produce doesn't depend on breast size. Big ones have more padding, but not necessarily more—or more effective—mammary glands. So relax, we know plenty of small-breasted women who've been successful at breastfeeding.

"When does breast milk form?"

A big hormone boost in your second trimester should already have your breasts producing milk and growing milk ducts (lobes in your mammary gland at the tip of your nipple). But, the milk factory won't actually kick into gear until after delivery. You'll start out with a thick, yellow fluid called colostrum, which is full of antibodies to help jump-start baby's immune system. There isn't a ton of it, but it's enough for baby's super-tiny tummy. On about day 3 or 4, your body should release the flood gates!

"Are my breasts going to start leaking before I even give birth?"

Maybe. Maybe not. First, colostrum will spring forth. It's possible to see it seeping out as early as the second trimester, or it may hold off until just after you deliver. Either way, you're fine and normal!

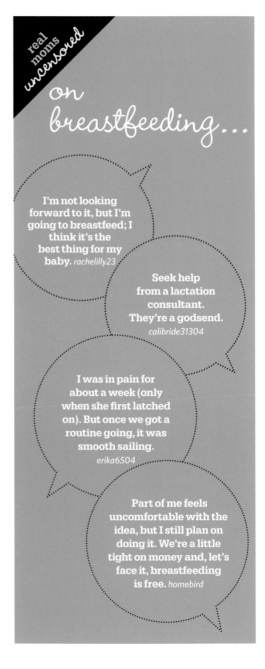

real moms *uncensored*

on breastfeeding...

I'm not looking forward to it, but I'm going to breastfeed; I think it's the best thing for my baby. *rachelilly23*

Seek help from a lactation consultant. They're a godsend. *calibride31304*

I was in pain for about a week (only when she first latched on). But once we got a routine going, it was smooth sailing. *erika6504*

Part of me feels uncomfortable with the idea, but I still plan on doing it. We're a little tight on money and, let's face it, breastfeeding is free. *homebird*

checklist

"what do I ask when I interview the pediatrician?"

Most importantly, you want to get a general feel for whether the doctor's personality, views, and communication style meshes with yours. You'll probably only have about 10 minutes to test the vibe, so ask questions that are most important to you first. Here are some to consider:

○ How long have you been practicing?

○ Do you have any sub-specialties?

○ What are your hours?

○ Do you offer same-day sick appointments? How far in advance do well appointments need to be scheduled?

○ What if my baby gets sick when the office is closed?

○ Is this a solo or group practice? If it's solo, who covers when you are gone? If it's a group, how often will we see you, and how often will we see others?

○ Do you have separate sick and well waiting rooms?

○ Do you respond to questions by e-mail? If I leave a message, how long does it usually take you to return the call?

○ Will your initial meeting with my baby be at the hospital or the first checkup? What is your schedule for well baby checkups?

○ Will you discuss general growth and issues like discipline and social development?

○ What are your views on . . . Bottle feeding? Circumcision? Parenting techniques? Getting babies to sleep? Alternative medicine? Antibiotics? Immunizations?

○ What hospitals do you work with?

○ Do you take my insurance? Is there an extra charge for . . . Advice calls during the day? Advice calls after hours? Medication refills? Filling out forms? Will any other fees apply?

○ What are your policies for insurance claims, lab policies, payments, and billing?

○ What tests are handled in the office, and what is done elsewhere? Where?

month 7

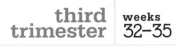
chapter 8

month

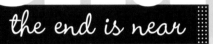
the end is near

eight

tick tock—baby will be here soon!

Your OB will probably start scheduling your appointments every two weeks at this point. Sure, you're falling asleep in meetings and wetting yourself pretty much whenever you sneeze, but who cares? You're about to be a mom! While baby kicks you in the ribs in the middle of the night, you're trying to come up with the perfect middle name. And wondering if you really need special infant laundry detergent. And how on earth you'll baby-proof an entire house. And if you'll ever have time to cook dinner again. And whether you're really the cloth diaper type. Oh, the list goes on and on!

your to-do list

• Have baby shower

• Pack your hospital bag

• Do some initial baby-proofing

• Cook a few meals to freeze

▶ Download our hospital bag checklist at TheBump.com/bag

what you're in for...

" I CAN'T BELIEVE MY BELLY WILL GET BIGGER THAN THIS!

Is this heavy discharge normal?

UGH...THE PRESSURE

difficult to breathe.

OMG—I JUST PEED WHEN I SNEEZED.

MY BELLY BUTTON POPPED.

ouch!

I'm obsessed with labor.

I'm sooo tired.

My feet barely fit in my shoes. "

on your mind...

▌at the ob's office

"What is the GBS test?"

For the Group B Strep (GBS) test, your OB will do a quick swab of your vagina and rectum with a big cotton swab, and then send the samples to a lab to check for a bacteria called group B streptococcus. From 10 to 30 percent of pregnant women carry GBS, even though most have never had symptoms. If you do have the GBS bacteria floating around—usually in your reproductive or digestive tracts—it can be passed to baby during delivery, possibly (but not always) leading to serious disorders or disabilities. If you test positive, you'll be treated with antibiotics during labor to keep baby in the

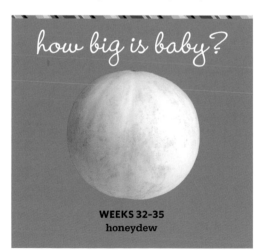

how big is baby?

WEEKS 32–35
honeydew

clear. Babies aren't exposed to GBS during c-sections, so antibiotics aren't necessary for planned cesareans. (You'll need to be tested anyway, though, in case you go into preterm labor.) Every woman should get this test between weeks 35 and 37, so ask your OB about it if she hasn't mentioned it yet.

"Will the doctor estimate baby's weight? How?"

Your OB may or may not venture a ballpark guess of baby's size. If she does throw out a number, don't expect it to be spot on. It's just a guesstimate, based on how big your uterus feels, how you're measuring, and your own stature. That said, many moms report being surprised by their doc's accurate guess!

▌in your head

"How can I be sure the baby will fit?"

While it seems like a tight squeeze, you aren't likely to have a baby that's larger than your body can handle. Biology just doesn't work that way. Generally speaking, if you're a tiny person, baby will end up on the small side too. Plus, your tissues have an incredible ability to stretch—and as long as baby can make it through the smallest part of your pelvic bones, you're golden. To help out, the bones of baby's skull don't harden and fuse together until after delivery, allowing for some squeezing and making baby's exit a little more streamlined.

"I've been put on bedrest! How do I keep from going insane with worry?"

First, the logistics. Decide where you'd like to set up camp (your bed? the couch?), and have your partner, mom, or friend create a

month 8

cozy, full-service nest for you. Stock it with a phone, plenty of reading material, paper and pencil, a TV with remote, lots of drinks and snacks (get a cooler for the perishable stuff), and a laptop with Internet access. Some moms like to alternate between mindless entertainment (Sudoku, daytime soaps) and baby preparations (pediatrician hunting, online shopping, making to-do lists for your partner). You can also use this time to take up a new hobby, like knitting or sketching. If your OB says it's okay, a little light exercise—like leg lifts—can get your blood flowing and keep you from feeling too sluggish. As for your emotions, try to find some support. It's normal to feel angry and worried when your pregnancy doesn't go according to plan. Share your feelings with your mate or a trusted friend. It can also help to connect with other moms-to-be who are also on bedrest—look for them in online mommy groups (like the third trimester message board on TheBump.com).

"Will my baby be breech?"

There's no way to know at this point if your baby will be one of the 3 to 4 percent of full-term babies who don't flip over into the head-down position. (And keep in mind that baby could still flip as late as week 39, 40 . . . or just before labor.) Most breech babies seem to simply be stuck in the wrong position (there isn't room to maneuver in your uterus these days), but there are a few risk factors that can contribute to a breech presentation. A few of these risk factors include:

- Too much or too little amniotic fluid
- Second (or further subsequent) pregnancy
- Multiples
- Abnormally shaped uterus and/or uterine growths (e.g., fibroids)
- Placenta previa (placenta covers some or all of the uterus's opening)
- Preterm birth
- Birth defects

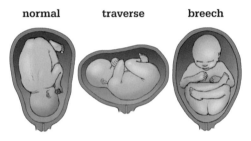

normal   traverse   breech

"When should I stop working?"

This one's really up to you. Some moms choose a "last day" a couple of days—or weeks—before their due dates in order to have a break before going into labor. Good for last minute shopping . . . and stocking up on sleep before parenthood. Other moms make arrangements to work from home in the final days. And lots of moms work right up until labor begins, saving every bit of maternity leave for after baby arrives. The bonus here: It keeps you from sitting at home begging for baby to hurry. Luckily, there is some evidence that you're more likely to go into labor at night, so odds are you won't be yelling, "This is it!" at the big budget meeting—though we can't promise. If you do plan to work right up to and possibly past your due date, just try to

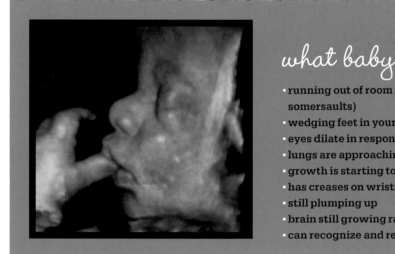

what baby's up to

- **running out of room (no more somersaults)**
- **wedging feet in your ribs**
- **eyes dilate in response to light**
- **lungs are approaching maturity**
- **growth is starting to slow**
- **has creases on wrists and neck**
- **still plumping up**
- **brain still growing rapidly**
- **can recognize and react to music**

tie up any major loose ends by the time you hit "full term" (37 weeks), so your colleagues have no reason to call in your first days with your new addition. Except to say "congrats!"

▍is it normal?

"My husband says I'm snoring now! Is this because I'm pregnant?"
Yes, pregnant women are more than twice as likely to snore as non-pregnant ones, and in the third trimester especially. Studies suggest that your new nighttime habit is due to more narrow upper airways, which should return to normal after delivery. There are also studies that link snoring in pregnancy to gestational diabetes, so it may be a good idea to let your OB know you're rattling the windows. And, as always, eat healthy and exercise (heavier women are more likely to snore). If you didn't snore before pregnancy, you'll probably return to silent snoozing after baby comes.

"I'm peeing a little every time I cough, sneeze, or laugh! What's going on?"
You bladder is shaped like a balloon with a little tube (your urethra) at the bottom to let out the urine. The muscles under your bladder usually keep that tube closed tight, but now there's a bowling ball of a baby pressing down on them, adding lots of additional pressure and putting those muscles to the test. And if they give way? Well, you leak pee. Don't worry, you've got a good defense: Kegels. In the meantime, a panty liner can at least help keep any leakage a secret.

month 8

▍delivery countdown

"What is my mucus plug? When can I expect it to come out?"

The "mucus plug" is the thick mucus your body uses to plug the opening of your cervix during pregnancy, sealing out bacteria and anything else harmful that could potentially make its way up to baby. You might see it come out (it can look like a glob of snot and is sometimes tinged with blood because tiny capillaries around it burst) in the last month of pregnancy, or you might not see it at all. (For some women, it comes out in pieces, or isn't very noticeable.) Your body will keep making mucus to fill its place, so you'll see a good deal of discharge from now until delivery. If your mucus plug comes out before week 36, give your OB a call—she might want to check you to make sure you aren't headed toward preterm labor. But if you see your mucus plug after that, don't get too excited—while it is definitely part of your body's prep for labor, it doesn't really predict when labor will come. (Could be hours later. Could be weeks.)

"Will I be able to tell the difference between losing my mucus plug and my water breaking?"

Many a first-time mom has confused these two, especially since a ton of discharge can follow the loss of your mucus plug. Think of it this way: Mucus is gooey; water is liquid. So if it's thick, it's not your water. When your water breaks, it will be like . . . water. Amniotic fluid will trickle or gush, and shouldn't have any color at all. It's possible, though, that the mucus will have a yellow, brown, or green tint—if so, be sure to let your OB know. This means baby has pooped and will need to be monitored in case she's breathed it into her lungs.

"What is back labor? Will I have it?"

With back labor, you feel discomfort (aka pain) in your lower back as labor progresses, usually right above your tailbone. Sometimes, back labor seems to set in if baby's head is pressing against your tailbone, or if baby is in an otherwise awkward position. But even if baby is perfectly aligned, you might not be in the clear. A few (unlucky) women simply tend to feel labor in their backs. Will you be one of them? There's no way to know until you go into labor. The experience of labor varies from woman to woman, and from pregnancy to pregnancy. If you do feel the pain, try standing under a warm shower, using hot or cold packs, having your mate massage you or apply pressure with his hands or a tennis ball, or changing positions. Of course, an epidural will do the trick, too.

"Is there anything I can do to avoid having a c-section?"

Not always. In most cases, they happen when your baby can't be delivered vaginally, no matter what you or your doctor does to help her along. For instance, you might need a c-section if your baby hasn't turned head-down in time for delivery, is especially large, or you have placenta previa.

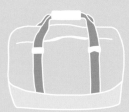

"what should I pack in my hospital bag?"

It's a good idea to have your bag ready by week 32. Here's what should be in it.

- Pairs of warm, nonskid socks that can get ruined
- Pajamas
- A warm robe or cardigan sweater
- 2 maternity bras—no underwire—and nursing pads (whether or not you plan to nurse)
- Lip balm (hospitals are very dry)
- Personal items like toothbrush, toothpaste, and deodorant
- Going-home clothes in 6-month maternity size and flat shoes

- Headband or ponytail holders
- Sanitary napkins. The hospital will provide, but you may prefer your own.
- Maternity underwear that can get ruined. You'll get some disposable pairs from the hospital which some women find handy and others find gross
- Music for the delivery room
- Going home outfit for baby
- Warm blankets (for the ride home)

- Insurance info, hospital forms and birth plan (if you have one)
- Sugar-free hard candy or lozenges to keep your mouth moist during labor (candy with sugar will make you thirsty)
- Pen and paper
- Very light reading (think magazines and newspapers)
- Diaper bag
- Car seat
- Camera, film or extra memory card, battery or charger

- Lots of change for the vending machines and non-perishable snacks (you'll probably be hungry after labor, and the hospital cafeteria could be closed)
- Cell phone and charger, phone numbers of people to call after birth, prepaid calling card (if your hospital doesn't allow cell phones)

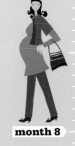

month 8

what to skip

- Jewelry
- Lots of cash
- Breast pump

- Medication (the hospital will provide)
- Diapers (ditto)

- Baby book (you won't have time or energy to write)

- Book to read (you probably won't have time or energy to read, either!)

Sometimes complications during labor force doctors to deliver a baby by c-section. If labor stalls (meaning that your cervix stops dilating); your baby's heart rate slows or becomes irregular; the umbilical cord slips through the cervix (a "prolapsed cord"); or the placenta separates from the uterine wall (placental abruption), your doctor will perform a c-section.

Try not to worry, though. Good prenatal care will boost your chances of delivering vaginally and handling any complications that arise. The important part is that baby gets here safely—no matter the route.

the day to day

"How do I decide between cloth and disposable diapers?"

The difference isn't as enormous as it used to be. Here's how they stack up:

HEALTH AND COMFORT No huge disparity, as long as you change baby's diaper when it's full (a little more often with cloth). Leaving on a soiled diaper increases risk of diaper rash and isn't too pleasant for baby. Your baby might prefer the softer feel of cloth diapers. Disposable diapers are more breathable, but their moisturizing, absorbent chemicals irritate some babies.

CONVENIENCE Forget the complicated folds and scary pins your mom had to deal with.

We always keep some disposables in the house for different things (I forget to do laundry, a bad rash, when we go out of town, etc.), but mainly use cloth diapers. *lily225*

Some cloth diapers come with Velcro or snap closures, fitted shapes, removable linings, and waterproof bands around the waist and legs, making the cloth change almost as quick and easy as the disposable. But cloth diapers aren't as absorbent, so you'll have to change them more often and do more laundry, or arrange for a diaper service.

PRICE Wash cloth diapers yourself and you'll save around $1,000 or more on your first child alone. The savings also depend on what sort of cloth diapers you purchase. (Prefolds are the least expensive option by far, while the sized, fitted—and cute!—versions can cost a pretty penny.) If you purchase second-hand diapers and/or save them for future children, your savings multiply. However, cloth diaper laundering services will set you back about the same amount as disposables—roughly $2,000 to $2,500 over three years.

ENVIRONMENT Not as clear cut as you might think. Yes, disposables use resources like trees and plastics during manufacturing, and then collect in landfills (most are 40 percent biodegradable). But consider the process of washing cloth diapers—clean water and energy are used, and nothing but dirty water is produced. (In other words, it's actually kind of a toss-up.) Note: For daycare or travel, disposables win hands down. Studies show they reduce infection risk in a group setting—in fact, many daycares don't allow cloth. Cloth is too inconvenient on the road.

"should I start with a bassinet rather than a crib?"

We know—you had one when you were little, your mother had one, your mother's mother had one . . . but unless you're getting a hand-me-down, it's probably not worth it since you'll likely only get a few weeks' worth of use out of it before it starts to collect dust in the corner of the room. Try a travel crib or even a play yard (many come with a bassinet option)—you'll get more use out of them later on. Spend your time now looking for a good, solid crib.

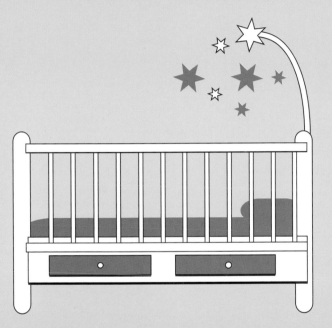

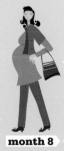

month 8

Even if you choose to start out with a bassinet or a bedside sleeper, every baby needs a crib eventually. A few rules:

- Follow the assembly directions.
- It should be 100 percent sturdy with no leftover pieces.
- Make sure slats are no more than 2⅜ inches apart so baby can't get stuck.
- The mattress should fit securely against the sides.
- Look for a lowering feature so the mattress can be moved down as baby grows.
- Only a waterproof pad and soft, fitted sheet are needed.
- Bumpers aren't necessary and can be a safety hazard (baby might get stuck under them and could suffocate).

"how do I baby proof my home?"

Baby won't be mobile for several months, but there are some things you can do to keep her safe in the meantime . . . and to prepare for the day when she does get moving!

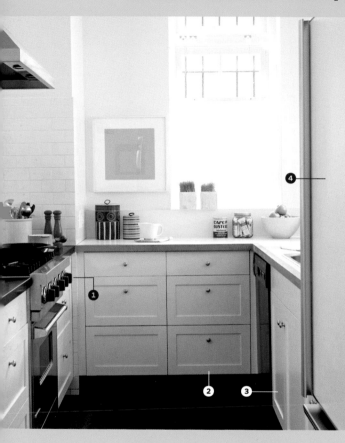

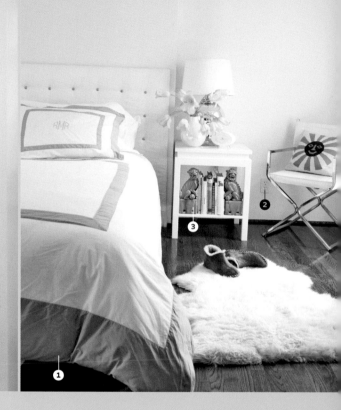

kitchen

1. Install stove guards and knob covers on oven.
2. Secure cabinets and drawers with latches.
3. Invest in a fire extinguisher; store in a cabinet near stove.
4. Move magnets off the fridge.

DON'T FORGET Use the back burners as much as possible and stow all cleaning items in high spots.

bedroom

1. Don't ditch your favorite duvet; cover with a sheet when baby's around.
2. Cover sockets with protectors.
3. Clear any exposed fragile items from nightstands.

DON'T FORGET Tame loose wires with cord clips and install window stops so windows open only 4 inches.

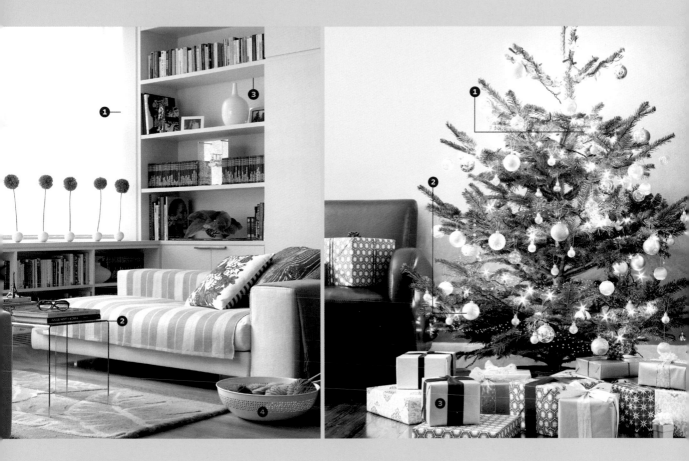

living room

1. Attach cord shorteners or wind-ups to window coverings.
2. Cushion sharp edges with guards.
3. Put brackets up high and out of reach.
4. Keep dangerous items off the floor.

DON'T FORGET Get a TV stand with a lip, to prevent it from tumbling over. Put a secure gate in front of a fireplace.

holiday

1. Choose lead-free lights.
2. Hang fragile ornaments on higher branches.
3. Keep wrapped gifts off the floor. Ribbons and bows are choking hazards.

DON'T FORGET At the holidays, skip holly, amaryllis, mistletoe, and tinsel; they're harmful if eaten.

real moms uncensored

on leaving work . . .

> My water started to leak while I was at work! *Senecamom*

> My last day at work was my due date. I went into labor the next day and didn't go in. I didn't want to lose a single day with my baby! *dnagal*

> I quit at the 6-month mark, knowing that I would not be returning to work and needing some time to myself before the baby came. It was the best decision I ever made. *MLE21707*

> I think that it is great to leave work a week or two early. Get a mani and pedi while you still can for goodness sake! *GigaGal*

"Do I need to wash all of baby's clothes before delivery?"

You should wash clothes (plus any blankets, sheets, and other fabrics) in dye- and scent-free detergent (skip the fabric softener and dryer sheets) before they come into contact with him to get rid of new-stuff chemicals that could irritate baby's virgin skin. But also think twice before tossing his full wardrobe in the washer. There's no way to know baby's size before delivery (or how quickly he'll grow), and you don't want to wind up with a closet full of clean, non-returnable outfits. Instead, wash a few of your favorites, and leave tags on the rest 'til you're positive that they'll be worn. (You can continue this tactic as baby grows—he may not fit into those cute 6-month duds when he's 6 months old.)

"I'm making my birth announcement list. Who do I send them to?"

At a bare minimum, send announcements to family and close friends. But feel free to include old friends, colleagues, close friends of your parents . . . anyone you think would be interested in your baby's birth. And don't worry that you're sending out too many. Birth announcements shouldn't make people feel pressured to send a gift (though you might receive a few "congrats" cards in the mail). They are simply pretty cards that let everyone know that baby has finally made an appearance. If you're keeping the mailing list small, you can cover the rest of the people with an e-mail announcement. (Just don't forget to attach a picture!)

"what should I look for in a baby monitor?"

After that first ride home from the hospital, the next scariest thing is probably putting baby to bed—away from you—for the first time. Monitors help you keep tabs through audio and/or video surveillance, giving you (relative) peace of mind.

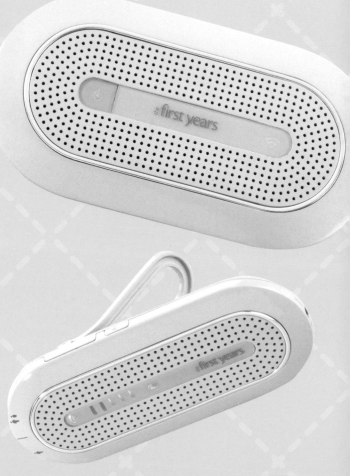

RECEIVERS This is what you hold onto to keep track of what's going on. Some are sold with one receiver, but you can buy a second.

SIZE If you have a big house, pick a monitor that's easy to carry around. Dorky as they are, belt clips can be very useful.

POWER SOURCE Some run on rechargeable batteries, some on regular ones, while others have a rechargeable base.

VIDEO FEATURES With these, you can watch what's happening (rather than just hear it) and potentially save yourself unnecessary trips to baby's room.

DIGITAL VS. ANALOG Digital monitors are pricier but they're better at limiting interference and protecting privacy (neighbors won't pick up sounds from your house on a wireless phone . . . or vice versa).

RANGE AND FREQUENCY How far will you want to travel from the nursery and still get reception? Many monitors sound an alert when you move out of range.

PAGING SYSTEM For when you inevitably misplace the receiver.

EXTRAS Night vision, Internet hookups so you can see baby while at work, the ability to pan and zoom, and sensor pads that go under baby's sheets and alert you if he stops moving (or breathing) are all great to have, but aren't necessary.

chapter 9

month

this is it—the final month & delivery!

nine

almost there now By week 37 or 38, you should be about as big as you're going to get (hallelujah), though baby will keep on growing straight through to delivery. Thirty-seven weeks also marks a "full term" pregnancy, meaning baby could show up any day and be expected to thrive! These last weeks can really drag on, but try not to lose it—no baby stays in forever. Just think, after all this fuss about pregnancy, now the real adventure begins. Soon you'll help baby find the way out of that giant belly and into your arms! Exciting, right? Here's the lowdown on what you're in for.

your to-do list

- Memorize the signs of labor

- Go on a date with your partner

- Make final preparations for baby

- Install the car seat

- Head to the hospital

Get more labor prep at
TheBump.com/delivery

what you're in for...

"

I'm peeing constantly.

There's suddenly more room between my belly and my boobs.

I was terrified I'd poop during labor... and when the time came, I SO didn't care.

TONS OF DISCHARGE.

I think this is it!

Come on, baby...

My belly itches like crazy.

I WANT TO CLEAN ALL THE WINDOWSILLS WITH A Q-TIP. TWICE.

WHERE DID THIS SUDDEN SURGE OF ENERGY COME FROM?

hurry up!

Now I really can't sleep.

PLEASE LET THIS BABY HAVE A TINY HEAD.

OMG— MY WATER BURST!

"

on your mind...

▌at the ob's office

"What is a nonstress test? And, why would I have one?"

The nonstress test (NST) checks in on baby's wellbeing by measuring how her heart rate responds to movement. (Just like yours, her heart rate should ideally speed up when she wiggles.) It's more likely that you will have a nonstress test if your pregnancy is high risk, or if you've gone past your due date. If your OB schedules you for this test, take a potty break first—it can last up to 40 minutes. You'll be hooked up to two devices, one to measure baby's heart rate and the second to record baby's movements. If baby is sleeping, the OB might use a (totally safe!) buzzer-like

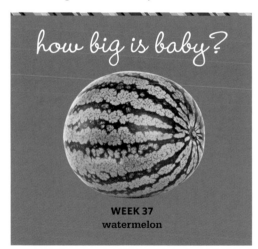

how big is baby?

WEEK 37
watermelon

instrument to wake her up. If baby's heart isn't speeding up when she moves, your OB might repeat the test or recommend either a contraction stress test or a biophysical profile, to make sure baby is okay in there.

"What's a contraction stress test?"

A contraction stress test is sometimes used to evaluate whether baby is in a strong enough condition to handle the stresses of labor. Most contraction stress tests are ordered to monitor the health of an overdue baby. If you have one, keep in mind that there is a fairly high rate of false positives (around 30 percent). How does it work? Basically, two different devices strapped around your belly will separately record fetal heart rate and contractions, while an IV drip of oxytocin causes your uterus to contract. (Sometimes there's no IV, and you'll be taught how to stimulate your nipples to naturally to coax the contractions instead.) If baby's doing fine, his heart rate will be constant, or will briefly dip during contractions and return to normal quickly. However, if his heart rate slows with contractions and stays that way, it might indicate fetal distress (usually due to a problem with the placenta), and your doctor may recommend an immediate c-section or induction of labor.

"What is a biophysical profile?"

Like the nonstress test and contraction stress test, a biophysical profile is often used to check on an overdue baby, or to evaluate a high-risk pregnancy in the third trimester. The test uses ultrasound to assess baby's body movement, muscle tone, breathing movements, and level of amniotic fluid, and is often combined with a nonstress test to add a heart-rate assessment into the mix. If all looks normal, your OB will probably

month 9

repeat the test once or twice a week until delivery. If not, she might schedule you for more tests (like the contraction stress test), or she might suggest delivering baby right away via induction or c-section.

"When will my OB start checking my cervix? Will she do it every time?"
Pelvic exams in pregnancy vary depending on the doctor and the practice. Your cervix's dilation and effacement might be checked every week starting at week 36 (or earlier!), or not until week 38 or 39, or your OB might not do a vaginal exam until you're in labor. Why? Well, the progress of your cervix doesn't always mean a lot, since it could dilate and efface slowly over the course of several weeks—or all at once on the day you deliver. If you go past your due date, however, your OB will almost definitely do an internal exam—the progress of your cervix (or lack of) can help her decide whether to consider induction. She might do an exam earlier if there is a specific concern, like bleeding or signs of preterm labor. If you're just curious about the status of your cervix and really want an internal exam, you can always request one. Don't be alarmed if you see some spotting afterwards—it's normal.

"How do I decipher what the OB tells me about my progress in an exam?"
Your doctor will use four measures to help evaluate your progress:
RIPENING is the softening of your cervix. The cervix must ripen before it can thin or open.

EFFACEMENT is the thinning of the cervix. This is measured in percentage, with 0 percent meaning no thinning has occurred yet and 100 percent being as thin as you'll get.
DILATION is the opening of your cervix. This is measured in centimeters, from 0 to 10. (Ten is when the cervix has stretched to the diameter of the largest part of baby's head.)
STATION is the position of baby's head as it relates to the ischial spines (bony spots on each side of the pelvis). It's measured on a scale of -5 (head floating above the pelvis) to +5 (head crowning at the vagina's opening).

"What is 'stripping your membranes'? Does it really get labor going?"
To "strip" your membranes, your doctor will sweep her (gloved) finger over the thin membranes that connect the amniotic sac and your uterus. This prompts your body to release prostaglandins, hormones that ripen the cervix and can bring on contractions. This procedure won't be done unless you go past your due date, and even then it isn't guaranteed to work.

in your head
"What if my OB isn't around on the day I go into labor?"
If you haven't asked your doctor who will deliver your baby in the case that she's not available, ask now. If you already have a good idea of who will be "on call" when your OB

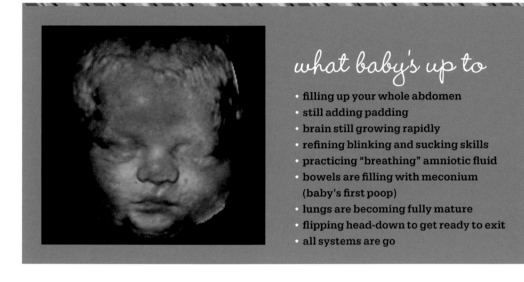

what baby's up to

- filling up your whole abdomen
- still adding padding
- brain still growing rapidly
- refining blinking and sucking skills
- practicing "breathing" amniotic fluid
- bowels are filling with meconium (baby's first poop)
- lungs are becoming fully mature
- flipping head-down to get ready to exit
- all systems are go

isn't and are simply panicking, settle down. Trust that your OB will leave you in good hands. Plus, you'll likely be spending more time with the labor nurses than with your OB.

"What if I think I'm in labor and the hospital sends me home?"

Well, you'll probably just get back in your car and go home. You might feel embarrassed, but the labor and delivery (or emergency room) staff are used to false alarms. Don't ignore labor symptoms for fear of being wrong, better to show up early than late!

"What if my due date goes right on by . . . but no baby?"

You won't be alone, that's for sure. Your due date isn't a deadline—it's more like an estimate. It's absolutely normal to go over, especially if this is your first baby. Go to your regularly scheduled OB appointments and try not to go nuts. Most OBs will schedule an induction if labor hasn't started by the time you hit 41 or 42 weeks. The end is in sight.

"I am SO ready for this kid to come out. Can I safely induce labor at home?"

Here's an answer you won't like: Not really. There are a few rumored remedies that you're welcome to try (taking a walk, eating spicy food, dancing, having sex), but don't get your hopes up that these will actually work. Other tactics (think: taking herbal supplements or castor oil, and stimulating your nipples) can do the trick, but we don't recommend them—they might bring on killer contractions that can be dangerous to your baby and super-painful to you. (Don't try these or any other methods without your midwife's or doctor's advice.)

month 9

▌is it normal?

"Why did I just feel like a lightning bolt shot through my vagina?"

This phenomenon doesn't seem very well documented, but we know many a mama who has complained of what we like to call "lightning crotch." What is it? Well, some women experience an occasional sharp pain in the pelvis or inside the vagina in the last weeks of pregnancy. This is probably related to your cervix dilating or to the pressure of baby's head on your cervix. (Either way, know that you're not alone.)

"I've heard moms talk about pooping during delivery? Is this common?"

Not everyone experiences this, but it's not at all unexpected. It's not usually very much, and the nurse just wipes it away. Trust us, it sounds like it would be humiliating, but you won't even care (or even necessarily know) when you're in the moment.

▌is it safe to . . .

"I'm full term anyway. Can I just ask the doctor to induce me already?"

Patience, child. Just because you are "full term" doesn't mean baby is ready to come out. Your body knows when the time is right, and it's safer not to cut it short, especially before you've passed your due date. Plus, induction isn't without risks. Inducing labor too early (for example, if your due

date projections were off) could result in a preterm birth, putting baby at risk for health issues. Induction also increases the risk of infection (for you and baby), umbilical cord problems, low fetal heart rate, the need for a c-section, and an increased risk of uterine rupture if you're trying for a VBAC (vaginal birth after cesaerean).

"Is it still okay for me to take a bath after my water has broken?"

There are different opinions on this one (some experts worry about risk of infection), so ask your OB or midwife to be sure. Once your water breaks, you shouldn't really do anything without running it by your doctor first. In fact, she'll probably want you to call as soon as the amniotic sac springs a leak, and will probably ask you to come on in to the hospital, at least in the next few hours.

▌delivery countdown

"What do contractions feel like? How much do they hurt?"

Since contractions are experienced slightly differently by different women, we can't really tell you. (Afraid we were going to say that, weren't you?) Some women describe contractions as feeling like super intense menstrual cramps; others of us feel a dull ache in our backs that wraps around to the front; and still others only feel a sharp pain in our backs, or only an intense pain in our bellies. Early contractions can also feel like a terribly upset stomach (diarrhea and all), or you might feel contractions radiating through your thighs. When asked to rate the degree of the pain, mamas-to-be also give drastically different answers, though the pain should always increase in intensity as labor progresses. And while chances are slim that this will be a near-painless experience (childbirth hurts—you knew that), you may be surprised to find the pain far easier—or yes, far tougher—to deal with than you're imagining. This pain has a purpose—you hurt because your uterine muscles are working hard to push baby into the world.

"How do I time contractions? Are there any tools to help?"

To time contractions, you'll pay attention to and record two things:

• The time each contraction begins
• How long each contraction lasts

This will tell you the frequency and duration of your contractions. (Note: To find out how "far apart" your contractions are, measure from the beginning of one contraction to the beginning of the next—NOT the time between them.) Your OB will probably give you a guideline for when to call or head to the hospital (like, when contractions are 5 minutes apart and lasting 30 to 45 seconds).

GREAT DEBATE

inducing labor: safe to stimulate?

natural labor is best

"When induction isn't necessary, it won't improve the labor outcome and can actually have the opposite effect. In our hospital, for women having their first baby, the c-section rate is 8 percent. If they're induced, it's 44 percent. If the woman's cervix isn't favorable and the baby isn't in a good position but you induce because of the calendar, you're inviting a c-section because you'll have a failed vaginal delivery." Dr. Michael C. Klein, MD, CCFP, FAAP (Neonatal-Perinatal), FCFP, ABFP

induction has benefits

"What I do is 'active management.' This means doing something about the risks rather than just simply waiting for something to happen. There aren't many situations where inducing can increase complications as long as you're aware of the cervical status. Plus, there's the added benefit of a scheduled delivery. If women can have elective c-sections, then why not elective inductions?" Dr. James M. Nicholson, MD

▶ Get more induction info at **TheBump.com/induction**

month 9

Keep track the old-fashioned way with a stopwatch and a piece of paper (if you're really in labor, you'll probably need your mate to help). Or, use an online contraction counter (we have one at TheBump.com/tools), and there are even a few iPhone applications that can help. Either way, you'll be looking for contractions that progressively last longer and come closer together. Each contraction might not be longer, or arrive sooner, than the one before it, but in true labor, a pattern will form over the course of a few hours.

"How can I tell if labor is coming soon?"

There's no real way to predict the moment (or even the week) that your body will post baby's eviction notice, but if you observe your body closely, you can tell preparations are underway in the days and weeks before labor hits. Here's what to look for.

NESTING Many women feel an overwhelming desire to clean and organize. The urges can be extreme (think scrubbing the bathroom grout with a toothbrush, or rearranging the living room furniture).

LIGHTENING This is when the baby "drops," settling down into your pelvis. You may or may not notice that your bump has changed shape, your lungs have more room (you can breathe again), and you feel the pressure of baby's head in your pelvis (beteen your legs) . . . and on your bladder.

DIARRHEA Many women experience diarrhea within a few days of labor, thought by some to be the body's way of emptying out before it needs to do all of that pushing.

STRONGER BRAXTON HICKS CONTRACTIONS Your "practice" contractions will probably get more uncomfortable within a couple of weeks of labor. (Remember: Real labor contractions will get consistently stronger, longer, and more frequent.)

LOSING YOUR MUCUS PLUG The mucus plug (see page 118) sometimes comes loose three or more weeks before delivery, but often just before true labor sets in. Either way, it means progress—your body is making way for baby.

A TON OF DISCHARGE After the mucus plug is expelled, you'll see a whole lot of clearish or whitish discharge.

BLOODY SHOW This pink-tinged discharge (as in blood from burst capillaries + the just-mentioned discharge) means your cervix has started to thin and/or dilate. Labor should be only days—or hours—away. (Call your OB immediately if you see bright red blood that looks like a period.)

YOUR WATER BREAKS There's a chance your membranes will rupture (meaning that the amniotic sac will burst or spring a leak) in the hours before labor begins. This happens for about 1 in 10 women. If you're one of them, call your OB to let her know! (If labor doesn't begin soon, you'll probably be induced.)

"How do I know if I'm in labor for real, or if it's false labor?"

When actual labor sets in, contractions get longer, stronger, and closer together—and they won't stop or decrease in intensity if you walk around or change position. You'll also see a bloody show (heavy discharge that's

chart

contraction counter

Think you're going into labor? Keep track of your contractions with our easy-to-use Contraction Counter. Or, try the digital one at TheBump.com.

	start time	stop time	length of contraction	frequency of contraction
1	:	:		
2	:	:		
3	:	:		
4	:	:		
5	:	:		
6	:	:		
7	:	:		
8	:	:		
9	:	:		
10	:	:		
11	:	:		
12	:	:		
13	:	:		
14	:	:		
15	:	:		
16	:	:		
17	:	:		
18	:	:		
19	:	:		
20	:	:		

month 9

pinkish or blood-streaked), and, of course, it's possible that your water will break.

With false labor, however, contractions won't be regular (you might have three that are 4 minutes apart, and then nothing for 20 minutes). They also won't get closer together or progressively more painful, and should ease up if you get up and walk, or change positions. You might also feel baby moving around during the contractions (but call your OB if baby seems frantic). If you see blood in false labor, it should be brownish (probably from an internal exam or from having sex in the past day or two).

"If I bleed during my last few weeks of pregnancy, am I going into labor?"
Maybe, but not always. If you're seeing blood-tinged mucus (aka "bloody show") along with other signs of early labor, like contractions, pressure in your pelvis or lower abdomen, or a dull lower backache, baby might be gearing up for arrival. However, light bleeding in late pregnancy could also be a sign of common conditions, like cervical growths or inflammation. Call your OB if you have any heavy red bleeding—this could signal a problem with the placenta, such as placental abruption or placenta previa.

"When will my water break?"
Imagining that scene in every movie and television show, where the woman's water breaks at the same instant that contractions set in? Don't count on this happening to you. Only about 10 percent of women have their membrane rupture before labor begins. So, you could be in that 10 percent, or your water could break sometime during labor, or your doctor might wind up breaking your water for you on the delivery table.

"What are my pain relief options for a vaginal delivery?"
There are several ways to lessen discomfort during labor and delivery.
SYSTEMIC ANALGESICS These are drugs that are injected into your muscle or a vein, and work on your whole nervous system to relieve (but not erase) your pain. They might make you tense or nauseated, so sometimes you'll receive another drug to relieve the side effects. Systemic analgesics are given more often early in labor—if given too close to delivery, baby can come out with slower reflexes and breathing.
EPIDURAL BLOCK An epidural block involves injecting analgesics (that numb you partially for a vaginal delivery) or anesthetics (that numb you more completely for a c-section, or if your OB needs to use forceps or a vacuum) into a space below your spinal cord known as the "epidural space." First, they'll numb you up with an injection of local anesthesia, and then the epidural needle is inserted. The anesthesiologist will probably thread a little tube through the needle and leave it in as a way to give you more epidural meds later in labor—or you might receive the drugs continuously. Your bottom half will be moderately numb within 10 to 20 minutes, and the degree of numbness can be adjusted.

on pain relief...

I wanted to go natural but I ended up being induced and the Pitocin was too much for me to take so I got the epidural. *ahnella*

It took them 7 attempts and I had a monster bruise afterward, but it was worth it! *MrsErinnElizabeth*

The epidural was a breeze going in. Didn't feel a thing getting it. I could still move my legs and was pretty mobile in bed. *dle927*

I was afraid of the epidural, but once I had it, I was in heaven. Three hours of pushing, forceps, and an episiotomy—I didn't feel a thing! Heaven! *krissyh21*

Epidural side effects include reduced blood pressure, shivering, and headaches. Rarely, the meds can enter a vein and cause a seizure or dizziness. They can also enter your spinal fluid and affect your chest muscles, making it hard to breathe (also rare).

SPINAL BLOCK A spinal block goes in through your lower back too, but with a much smaller needle, and your lower half is instantly numbed. It lasts only an hour or two, so you probably want to save it up for pushing time. Side effects are the same as with an epidural.

COMBINED SPINAL-EPIDURAL BLOCK Also known as a "walking epidural," the combined block is injected into both the spinal fluid and the space below the spinal cord. You'll have instant relief, and can have more drugs through the epidural for pain relief all the way through delivery. And yes, you might be able to walk around once the block is in place.

LOCAL ANESTHESIA Local anesthetics won't help your contractions, but they can be injected to numb a small area (like your perineum before an episiotomy or stitches).

GENERAL ANESTHESIA General anesthesia knocks you out cold. You probably won't receive this unless you wind up needing an emergency c-section and spinal block or epidural isn't possible or practical for some reason. If you need to be put under, the meds will cause you to lose consciousness quickly, and the anesthesiologist will put a breathing tube down your windpipe after you're out.

ALTERNATIVE THERAPIES If you'd rather skip the meds, you may find relief through self-hypnosis, soaking in water, transcutaneous

month 9

electrical nerve stimulation (or TENS—a therapy using little electrical jolts to reduce pain), meditation, or Lamaze.

"I'm scheduled for a c-section, and am nervous about the anesthesia. What are my options?"
For a c-section, the choices are an epidural block, a spinal block, or general anesthesia. You may or may not have a choice—your OB may take your preferences into account, but she'll ultimately make a decision based on both your and baby's well-being. If you're put under general anesthesia, you won't be awake for the cesarean. With the epidural and spinal blocks, the lower half of your body will be numbed for the surgery, but you'll remain awake. Try not to worry about it too much. Yes, all three anesthesia options will involve a needle, but the needle prick is guaranteed to be less painful than what you'd feel without it! Women have c-sections every day—and no matter how you're numbed, you'll be meeting your baby in no time.

"How should my baby be positioned?"
Ideally, your little one will be head down— probably facing your side for now—and will come out facing your back. Her head will

GREAT DEBATE

circumcision . . . should you snip?

foreskin should stay
"Circumcision is unnecessary, risky, traumatic, and harmful. Also, all of the 'health' reasons for getting one have been debunked. It's painful, and the emotional trauma is stored deep in the brain. Severe bleeding can occur, and every year babies actually die from the procedure. Plus, there are chronic complications that might appear later, erectile dysfunction for one. Many people feel that it violates human rights." *Dr. Mark D. Reiss, MD*

snip the skin
"Circumcision is a very valuable preventative measure. A male who's uncircumcised has 10 times the risk of contracting a urinary tract infection during the first year of his life (when they're most dangerous). He's 3 times as likely to get HPV, which causes penile and cervical cancer. In fact, nearly 100 percent of penile cancer cases are in uncircumcised men." *Dr. Edgar Schoen, MD*

▶ Weigh in on snipping at **TheBump.com/circumcision**

duck as she descends through the birth canal, so she'll come out crown-first. (Hence the cone-head look that new babies tend to sport.) This position makes for the easiest, most streamlined delivery.

"What is a version?"

A cephalic version is basically when your OB pushes and prods your breech baby to try and get him to turn head-down (a technique some doctors use to try and shift a baby into the proper birthing position). First, they'll do an ultrasound to determine baby's position, heart rate, the placenta's position, and the amount of amniotic fluid. You might also be given a medicine to relax your uterus and ease the turning. Next, the doctor (and maybe a helper) will push or lift your tummy with his hands to try and help baby roll into position. She might use ultrasound to guide her in the procedure, and to keep track of baby's heart rate. Your doctor isn't likely to attempt a version until after 36 weeks, since baby is still likely to turn a somersault before then. And yes, even if your OB does manage to get baby into position, he could still flip right back into his favorite spot. The good news: More than half of version attempts are successful—so it's definitely worth a shot. Complications from a version are rare, but you'll probably have the procedure done in or near a delivery room, so that baby could be delivered quickly in the

My first baby was breech until about 30–31 weeks, he turned on his own and I totally felt it when he did. They can flip-flop until there isn't enough room in there. *lkf041*

(unlikely) case of early membrane rupture, heart rate problems, placental abruption, or preterm labor.

"Anything I can do to get baby to turn?"

Unfortunately, there's no surefire way to make baby shift. If there were, we would rarely see breech babies. Still, there are a couple of things you can try. (These aren't necessarily proven effective, but they aren't total hogwash either—both methods have seemed to turn a number of fetuses in scientific studies.)

KNEE-CHEST POSITION Get on your hands and knees (in a crawling position) on the bed, and lay your head, shoulders, and chest flat on the mattress. If your belly is pressed against your thighs, scoot your knees back until it's hanging free. Hold for 15 minutes, and repeat every two hours while awake.

MOXIBUSTION Acupuncturists experienced in turning breech babies may be able to urge baby to flip by burning an herb—moxa, aka mugwort—near your little toe. (Nope, we're not kidding.)

"My baby still is breech—I'm definitely going to have a c-section, right?"

Most OBs will recommend a cesarean, but a vaginal birth might still be an option, too, especially if a version (turning the baby manually) is successful. When your due date nears and baby is still breech, you and

month 9

your OB will inevitably discuss both the risks and benefits of giving a version—or even a breech delivery—a shot.

"How come most breech babies are delivered by c-section?"
Well, a vaginal breech delivery can be pretty tough. Baby's head is the largest part of his body. When it comes out first, it stretches the cervix enough that the rest of the body comes out fairly easily afterwards. However, if the body comes out first (as with a breech baby), it might not stretch the cervix enough for the larger head to fit. In a vaginal breech birth, a prolapsed umbilical cord—when the cord goes through the birth canal before baby—is also more likely. A prolapsed cord can become pinched, which cuts off blood flow (and puts baby in serious danger).

8 or 9 years. (Sex almost definitely won't happen for 6 weeks.) Cook together or order in and cuddle in the living room.
DOUBLE DATE Go out with your childless couple-friends and pack in adult interaction before the little one takes over. And try not to talk about the baby. No, you two won't be alone, but you can use this as a time to reconnect with your partner as a person (as opposed to a babymaker).

"Does it really matter if I keep eating healthy and exercising at this point?"
You have every right to take it easy in these last weeks of pregnancy, but keep in mind that keeping up your healthy habits can serve to make you more comfortable. And, staying moderately active and eating right can keep your swelling down, your energy up, and, of course, better equip you for baby's arrival.

▍the day-to-day

"Any tips for a final date night? I guess we won't have another for awhile!"
You're right that time alone with your spouse can be scarce in the first weeks (or years) with baby. Make the most of your final few evenings together before becoming parents.
CATCH A FLICK There are lots of places where you can bring an infant. A movie theater is not one of them. See a blockbuster on the big screen before you're doomed to Netflix.
HAVE A CANDLELIT DINNER A romantic evening at home might not happen for the next, oh,

▍the big day

"What will happen when I get to the hospital or birthing center?"
The exact routine depends on your hospital's specific procedures, but odds are good that it will go something like this: First, you'll check in. (If you pre-registered, this will only take a second.) Next, you'll either have the dilation of your cervix checked in a triage room (to make sure you're really in active labor), or you'll be taken to your labor or birthing room

"can you help me understand the stages of labor?"

Sure. There's a lot that happens, and no two labors are the same, but here's the status quo:

stage 1

This stage is the longest and is divided into three phases of its own.

EARLY LABOR Your cervix effaces (thins) and dilates from 0 cm to 3 cm. Mild to moderate contractions set in, coming every 5 to 20 minutes and lasting 30 to 60 seconds.

TO DO
- Rest or nap
- Have a light snack
- Pee frequently (a full bladder slows labor)
- Double-check your hospital bag
- Time contractions

ACTIVE LABOR Your cervix opens from 3 cm to 7 cm. Your contractions get more intense, coming every 3 to 4 minutes and lasting 40 to 60 seconds each. You'll head to the hospital as this phase begins.

TO DO
- Practice your breathing exercises
- Try to relax between contractions
- Keep peeing at least once an hour
- Walk around if you can
- Get pain relief, if you want it

TRANSITION Your cervix dilates to 10 cm. Contractions will last 2 to 3 minutes and come every 60 to 90 seconds.

TO DO
- Use your breathing exercises
- Don't push until your OB says to
- Try to stay focused

stage 2

This stage begins when you're fully dilated. Contractions will probably stay around 60 to 90 seconds, but may be further apart (usually 2 to 5 minutes). You'll want to push.

TO DO
- Breathe—your baby needs your oxygen
- Try to stay (relatively) calm and focused
- Concentrate on relaxing any tense body parts
- Get into a position that uses gravity to your best advantage
- Go with the flow—your body knows what to do
- Rest between contractions
- Ask for a mirror if you want to see just what is happening down there
- Push with all your might!

stage 3

After baby arrives, your uterus will contract again (mildly) to kick out the placenta. This lasts about 5 to 10 minutes, but can take up to 30. Once that's out, your OB will stitch up any tears or your episiotomy, and labor is done!

TO DO
- Push if the doctor asks you to
- Thank your coach for the support
- Relax and enjoy your baby

month 9

and admitted—you'll be having a baby today! Once in the room, you'll be quizzed about your status (when your contractions started, how far apart they are, if your water has broken), given a lovely butt-baring hospital gown to change into, and asked to sign a few routine consent forms. Once you hop (okay, maybe not hop, exactly) onto the bed, the nurse will check your vitals (pulse, blood pressure, temperature, breathing), check your cervix if you weren't checked in triage, look for anything leaking out of you (like blood or amniotic fluid), and check baby's heart rate with a Doppler or fetal monitor. She'll check baby's position too. You may be hooked up to IV fluids at this point (this is routine in some hospitals, but not in others), and you may also be hooked up to external or internal fetal monitors, depending on the hospital and doctor's policies, the risk level of your pregnancy, and baby's status. (Intermittent monitoring with the Doppler might be allowed instead, especially if you'll be walking around in labor. Talk to your OB if this is what you'd prefer.)

"Will the doctor break my water?"
If your water (aka "amniotic sac," "bag of waters," or "membranes") hasn't broken on its own when you arrive at the hospital, and you're 5 or more centimeters dilated, your OB might recommend bursting the bag by hand—especially if your cervix seems to be making slow (or no) progress. (Some OBs will go ahead and break your water at 3 or 4 centimeters.) The reasoning behind this:

"Artificial rupture of membranes" (popping a hole in the amniotic sac) will usually jump-start labor by getting serious contractions underway. If labor is moving along fine, you and your doctor might decide to wait this one out—after all, contractions tend to be more painful after your water breaks. If the OB doesn't rupture your membranes, the sac will probably break on its own during labor, though once in a while it stays intact until baby makes an exit. (Either way is fine.)

To break your water, the doctor will reach up and prod it with something that looks like a crochet hook. You might feel (very little) discomfort as the device enters your vagina, but as for the actual water breaking, most women only feel a big, warm gush of liquid.

"How will they make sure my baby is okay during labor?"
DOPPLER If your pregnancy is low risk and baby has been doing A-okay so far, your OB or nurses might simply keep tabs on baby's heart rate with a Fetal Doppler monitor (the same way they listen to baby at your prenatal appointments). If that's the case, they'll probably check in at least every half-hour before you start pushing, and then every 5 minutes during delivery.
EXTERNAL FETAL MONITOR Intermittent monitoring can be time consuming, you might have a fetal monitor strapped to your bump instead. (This is routine in many hospitals.) The monitor consists of two small devices, one that tracks your contractions, and one that tracks baby's heartbeat. Both

delivery room

headwalls Just behind the bed on the headwalls you will find the nurse call system, oxygen, suction, and air for you and baby.

hemodynamic monitor This monitor measures your heart rate, blood pressure, and O^2 saturation.

fetal monitor A strap will be placed around your belly with two monitors—one tracks baby's heart rate; the other tracks your contractions.

radiant heat warmer This device helps to keep baby's temperature regulated after birth and during the initial assessment.

bed The entire bottom drops out and the stirrups come up when it's time to deliver. The bed might also have handlebars to hold onto as you push.

patient care cart This holds all the supplies needed for labor including peri-pads, IV supplies, gauze and slippers.

partition To give you privacy during the actual birth and to block off what's going on outside your room if you need to rest during a long labor.

will be hooked to a monitor that will print out the data or display it on a screen (the same info may be on display for doctors or nurses down the hall). You may have these strapped around you during the whole labor.

INTERNAL FETAL MONITOR If your doctor feels the need to keep a closer watch on baby's status (especially if she thinks baby may be in distress), she may reach up and stick an electrode on baby's head. (Clearly, you'll have to be a little dilated first, and your water must be broken.) The electrode tracks baby's heart rate, and you may also have a little tube (aka catheter) stuck into your uterus to gauge the contractions. Sometimes they skip the catheter and monitor contractions with the external device on your tummy. There are a few small risks involved, like irritation or infection, or sometimes even an abscess or, rarely, a bald spot where the electrode is placed, so you won't have an internal monitor unless there is a clear need for it.

"I don't remember anything from my hospital tour. What should I know?"

Hospitals vary in their delivery room setup— some will keep you in one room the entire time, while others have a room specifically for delivery, and then will move you to a separate recovery room. Some hospitals have delivery rooms specially designed to be comfortable and soothing, while others feel more like . . . well . . . hospital rooms. It's a very good idea to take a tour before you go, so that you feel comfortable and you're prepared for whatever your situation is.

"What are some good positions to try to make labor easier?"

Different positions feel different to different women, so experiment to find what feels right for you. That being said, here are some tried and true ones:

GET DOWN ON YOUR HANDS AND KNEES This position is good for relieving back labor.

HAVE YOUR PARTNER SIT IN A CHAIR WITH HIS LEGS APART Stand between his legs with your butt facing him, and go into a squat with your thighs spread apart (imagine making room for baby). Then, drape your arms over his knees to support yourself, and ask for a shoulder massage.

STAND FACING YOUR PARTNER, WITH YOUR ARMS AROUND HIS NECK Lean into him, or hang from his shoulders, and sway. This uses gravity to your advantage, gives you a break so that you don't have to hold all your own weight, and the movement helps get you through some seriously painful contractions.

LIE ON YOUR LEFT SIDE This is a great way to rest between contractions, and maximizes blood (and oxygen) flow to baby.

"Why do I need an IV during labor?"

For the most part, an IV is put in place so that there is a way to immediately plug any medicines into your blood stream if it becomes necessary. Your OB might also use a drip of IV fluids to keep you hydrated during labor. (Just in case any medicines are ordered without your knowledge, always ask what is being sent through your IV line, or have your labor coach read the bag.)

"what exactly are these tools and how are they used?"

Don't be alarmed when you see a nurse don a sterile hat, mask, and gloves—this means you're getting close to delivery and it's time to set up the doctor's table, nothing's suddenly gone wrong. The nurse is simply keeping things sterile. Here's what's being set up:

forceps We admit, they look a little scary. These are generally used to try and shift baby's position, and may also help guide the head out.

vacuum If pushing is proving ineffective, your doc will use this to pull the baby out with suction. Don't be alarmed.

hemostat This clamp is used to for containing any type of bleed, holding sutures, and—most importantly—cutting baby's umbilical cord.

amniotic hook It looks a lot scarier than it feels, we promise. This long crochet-like hook is used in the early stages of delivery to break your water if it hasn't yet happened naturally.

scalpel Unless you're having a c-section, your doctor probably won't use this—but it's kept on hand.

scissors Just in case you (Sorry! Really!) need an episiotomy.

you'll also see

SPONGE HOLDERS These rings are simply used to hold gauze.

LAPAROSCOPIC SPONGES If you start to bleed, your doc will hold these down to control it.

BUCKETS OF STERILE WATER Used to keep everything clean throughout the delivery.

SUTURES Your doc will use these to stitch you up if you tear or have an episiotomy.

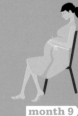

month 9

"What does it mean if the doctor says I have a 'lip' left when she checks me?"
Basically, this term means that you're fully dilated, but an edge of your cervix (usually the anterior—or front—of the cervix) is a little bit swollen and is still in the way of baby's head. Your OB may wait until it moves into the correct position on its own, or she may try to pull it out of the way with her fingers while you bear down to push the baby past. Just be sure to wait until your doctor gives the okay to push—pushing against an anterior lip can make the swelling worse . . . and make it more difficult to get baby out.

"What is a prolapsed cord?"
A prolapsed cord is when the umbilical cord manages to get in the way of baby's exit and slips into the birth canal first—usually when the water breaks. Baby can push against the cord during labor, compressing it so that less oxygen is making its way to your little one. This is very dangerous for baby, and might require an emergency c-section. If you think you can feel the cord in your vagina after your water breaks, get on your hands and knees (to reduce as much pressure on the cord as possible) in the back seat of the car while someone rushes you to the hospital, or call 911. Your doctor will most definitely want to get baby out right away.

Prolapsed cords are more likely to occur with premature labors or with breech vaginal deliveries, but they are very rare (about 1 in 1,000 deliveries), so your chances of having to deal with this are slim.

"Should I be worried about the cord wrapping around baby's neck?"
The umbilical cord winds up around a baby's neck in about 25 percent of deliveries. (It's called a "nuchal cord.") Most of the time, it stays pretty loose and causes no harm. Your OB will simply use a finger to slip the cord over baby's head at birth, or will clamp and cut it if it's wrapped too snugly. Occasionally, though, this can be dangerous (if it gets wrapped or knotted so tightly that it cuts off baby's blood supply). A decrease in fetal activity (keep up your kick counts and call your OB if you notice them slowing down) or an abnormal heart rate during labor are signs of a troublesome nuchal cord. The same goes for other tangles or knots that sometimes form in the cord.

"What will the placenta and umbilical cord look like when I deliver them?"
The umbilical cord looks like a flexible, spongy, twisted tube, consisting of two arteries and a vein covered in a whitish, see-through jelly. The placenta can be described as "cake-like," and is also spongy. It's big, bloody, veiny, and lumpy, with one red side (the side that was attached to your uterus) and one gray or silver side (the side that faced baby for all those months).

"What is an episiotomy? Is it likely that I'll have to have one?"
An episiotomy is an incision in the perineum (the skin between the vagina and anus) that helps baby fit through. Some OBs routinely perform episiotomies to make way for

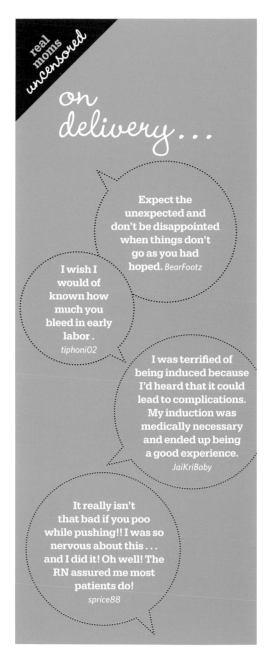

real moms uncensored

on delivery...

Expect the unexpected and don't be disappointed when things don't go as you had hoped. *BearFootz*

I wish I would of known how much you bleed in early labor. *tiphoni02*

I was terrified of being induced because I'd heard that it could lead to complications. My induction was medically necessary and ended up being a good experience. *JaiKriBaby*

It really isn't that bad if you poo while pushing!! I was so nervous about this ... and I did it! Oh well! The RN assured me most patients do! *sprice88*

baby, and others feel that it's better to tear naturally (though hopefully you won't tear at all!). Fewer episiotomies are performed these days, but most OBs will still perform an episiotomy in certain situations, such as to help deliver baby more quickly when there are signs of fetal distress, or if she'll need to use the forceps or vacuum extractor.

If your doctor does decide you need an episiotomy, you'll receive a local anesthetic (unless your perineum is already numb from the pressure of baby's head, or from an epidural). Then your OB will make a small slice in your perineum, usually either straight down towards your anus, or angled to the side. Once baby is safely delivered, you'll get another shot of local anesthesia (you'll feel a pinch) and a few stitches, which should disintegrate in a matter of weeks.

"In what scenario might I have to have an emergency c-section?"

In general, emergency c-sections are called for if anything happens to put you or baby in danger, like a prolapsed cord (umbilical cord coming out ahead of baby), placental abruption (the placenta starts coming loose, causing you and baby to loose blood), a breech presentation (baby isn't head-down for delivery), or fetal distress. You might also wind up with an emergency c-section if your labor stops progressing or takes way too long, especially if it has been several hours since your membranes ruptured (once he isn't surrounded by the amniotic sac, baby is susceptible to infection).

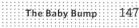

month 9

"What happens during a c-section?"

Whether your cesarean is scheduled ahead due to complications or baby's position (or yes, even personal preference), or you're wheeled into the OR for an emergency c-section, the basics are the same:

First, a nurse will prep you for the surgery. This entails washing (and maybe shaving) your abdomen, and you might be given medication to reduce stomach acid so that it doesn't enter your lungs. You'll also receive an IV in your arm or hand, to pump you with any meds and fluids during the procedure. A catheter (a thin plastic tube) will be put in your bladder to empty it during surgery, which lowers your risk of injury, and you'll receive anesthesia (either an epidural, a spinal, or general anesthesia—see page 136). Oh, and you get to wear a hair net. (Are you brimming with excitement yet?)

In most cases, your partner will be able to join you for the surgery—he'll just have to wash up and don a snazzy set of sterile scrubs beforehand, along with a mask and hair net. And don't worry about getting squeamish—you'll probably have a little curtain across your chest, blocking your view of all the exciting action.

Once you're under (or numbed), the OB will make either a vertical or transverse (aka horizontal) incision above your pubic hairline, going through your skin and abdomen. (The muscles can be moved, so, in most cases, they don't need to be cut.) Then, another incision— again either vertical or transverse—is made in your uterine wall. Because they're done on the lower, thinner part of the uterus and thus you'll bleed less and heal better, transverse incisions are usually the first option. However, in some specific circumstances, such as a very preterm baby not yet in the head-down position, a vertical incision may be necessary.

Next comes the fun part: The doctor will gently pull your baby out through these incisions! Just after delivery, the doctor (or your partner) will cut the umbilical cord, and the placenta will be removed. Your uterus will be closed with dissolvable stitches, and more stitches or staples will close up your skin. You may or may not get to hold your baby for a few seconds—depending on the baby's perceived health (and whether you're conscious)—but, barring any major health issues, you'll soon meet again the recovery room where you can begin ooh-ing and aah-ing over your bundle of joy.

"What will my baby look like when he finally comes out?"

Sure, all newborns are beautiful miracles. But as far as aesthetics go, well, they tend to look like little larva that just squeezed through a tight, slimy tube after soaking in fluid for 9 months. If baby is born vaginally, he might have a cone-head (c-section babies don't usually suffer this fate). And no matter the exit route, baby is likely to be wrinkly and might have swollen genitals and breasts, a coating of cheese-like vernix caseosa, a little fur (lanugo) on his back and head, poofy eyes, scratches, rashes, and other blotches and skin weirdness. But don't worry—he'll

"what medical staff will be in the room when I deliver?"

Good question—it's nice to be prepared for who'll be hanging around (and staring at your naughty bits) when you're in the delivery room. Hospitals have varied policies on what staff is present, but here's a rundown on the basics.

LABOR AND DELIVERY NURSE Your line of communication with your delivery practitioner and your support system. She's the one who monitors your progress and checks on baby as you dilate. You might have the same nurse for all of labor, or there could be one or more switches in staff due to shift changes.

DOCTOR OR MIDWIFE This is the person who delivers your baby. It may or may not be the one that you've been seeing throughout your pregnancy (for example, your OB may be on vacation on the day you go into labor or be part of a practice that rotates which doctor is on call on each day).

ANESTHESIOLOGIST If you'll receive pain relief during labor (spinal, epidural, or other meds), an anesthesiologist and/or nurse anesthetist may be present to drug you up.

OB TECH Sometimes an OB Tech will come in just before delivery to assist the doctor or midwife and set up any instruments.

OTHER NURSE(S), SPECIALISTS, STUDENTS Depending on the hospital and the circumstances that surround your birth, there may be other staff present, like a nursery nurse, neonatologist, or medical student. You might also choose to have a doula present to offer emotional support.

month 9

be gorgeous in his own way, and will come to look much more like a chubby Gerber baby in a couple of months time.

"What is an APGAR score?"

At 1 minute and again at 5 minutes after birth, the medical staff will evaluate your baby's activity and muscle tone, pulse, grimace response (ability to get mad), appearance (skin color), and respiration. They'll give each of these a score from 0 to 2 (with 2 being the best score) and then add those numbers together. The point of the APGAR scores is to check whether baby needs immediate medical care. Generally, a score over 7 is considered healthy. A lower score means baby might need special attention—or she may just need a little time. No need to mention baby's APGARs on her chic birth announcements—the test is a tool for your doctors and isn't meant to have anything to do with baby's future health, intelligence, or behavior. Your doctor will let you know if there is any cause for concern.

"What will happen to my baby in the hours after delivery?"

The routine differs depending on the hospital and doctor, but it usually goes something like this: Once baby is out, your OB will clamp and cut (or let your partner cut) the cord. (Baby will probably be lying on your tummy or chest for this.) Next, they'll check his APGAR scores, give baby a good rubdown with a towel, weigh and measure him, and give you and baby matching wrist and/or ankle bands. Baby will

also get eye ointment to prevent infection, and will probably be wrapped up really tight to keep warm. You'll probably get to cuddle with your new addition for awhile, and you may be able to give breastfeeding a go. (Baby may or may not be ready to eat right away though.)

After you've smothered your wee one in kisses (and taken a million pictures), baby will probably head to the newborn nursery for his first bath, his first pediatrician visit (for a thorough checkup), footprints (if they weren't taken in the delivery room), a routine heel stick (for government-required blood work), a hepatitis B shot, and possibly other protective procedures. You partner may be able to join baby for the whole deal—just ask. If all is well, baby will be deposited back in your arms once he's fully evaluated and swaddled up nice and tight.

"How long will I stay in the hospital?"

If you have a totally smooth vaginal birth, you're likely to head home within 24 to 48 hours of delivery. You'll have to wait for any anesthesia to wear off, rest a bit after all that pushing to get baby out, and, your OB may want to monitor you and baby for the first day or so to make sure no problems develop. Then, if all is well, you're likely to be back in your pad in no time.

Keep in mind that you may need to stick around for awhile if you have a cesarean or any complications. Use your extra time in the hospital to get some sleep and make sure to take advantage of the available support, like breastfeeding and baby care classes.

"I'm confused by some things in the bag the nurse just gave me. what are they?"

While it's probably the least sexy goody bag you'll ever receive, the loot your hospital sends you home with will definitely come in handy. Who doesn't love freebies? Every hospital is different in what they send you home with, but you should get most of these items.

peribottle Fill the peribottle with warm water, and squirt it on yourself as you go to the bathroom. It's also good for relieving itchiness when you can't scratch.

super-thick pads You'll still have a very heavy flow after you give birth, so heavy-duty pads are a necessity.

donut pillow Sitting down ain't easy in the days following delivery, but this round, open pillow will certainly help.

skin numbing spray If you have a tear or episiotomy, this will help with the pain.

witch hazel pads Whether or not you have hemorrhoids, these will help sooth your entire tender area. Chilling them may provide even more relief.

sitz bath This sits over your toilet and allows you to soak your delivery area in warm water, causing more blood to flow there to promote healing.

disposable mesh undies They also help keep your heavy-duty pads in place. Some moms love the disposable undies for their convenience.

"Puppy pad" These waterproof pads can be placed under you while you sleep, just in case. If you don't need them, use them for baby's changing table.

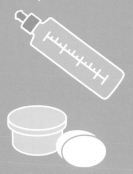

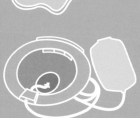

you'll also see

PAIN MEDS If you needed a c-section or had a complicated delivery.

INSTRUCTION BOOKLET No matter how many parenting books you have, the hospital booklet is always good to reference for advice about both your recovery and your newborn.

RESOURCE LISTS Information about support groups and other new-mom resources.

month 9

chapter 10

month

now what do I do with this thing?

ten

you made it through pregnancy—and delivery. It's over! . . . Actually, of course, it's only just beginning. Now you have to figure out motherhood: the feeding, the bathing, the breastfeeding, the diaper-changing, and, oh . . . the sleeping! Relax, you'll get the hang of everything. Eventually, you'll know what to do for baby better than anyone in the world. Just don't freak out if adjusting to this new life doesn't "come naturally"—it's a little bit tougher for some than it is for others. These first few weeks are a time for resting, recovering, and getting to know your babe as you and your guy figure out how to navigate life with this amazing new addition to your family!

your to-do list

- Schedule postpartum appointment
- Schedule baby's first checkup
- Track baby's feedings
- Keep up with your Kegels

Check out even more new mom advice at TheBump.com/newborn

what you're in for...

"**All this blood really freaks me out!**

SO CUTE ... SO LITTLE.

Everything hurts!

I CAN'T STOP CRYING.

Are you sure I can keep this tiny creature alive?

I hope my nipples get used to this breastfeeding thing soon.

I'm so overwhelmed!

Engorgement sucks!

PEOPLE KEEP ASKING IF THERE'S ANOTHER BABY IN THERE. YES, I'M STILL HUGE. THANKS.

MAN, PUSHING REALLY BEAT ME UP—I LOOK TERRIBLE!

I am terrified to poop!"

on your mind...

▎care basics

"When will I need to take baby to the pediatrician for the first time?"

Most pediatricians will want to see baby at least at birth, 2 to 4 days after birth, and then at 2, 4, 6, 9, and 12 months, the minimum recommended by the American Academy of Pediatrics. Every doctor's preferences are different, though, and some ask to see babies more often. Talk to yours to see what sort of schedule to expect.

"How do I care for the umbilical cord stump?"

The recommendations for this have changed a lot in recent years, and not all doctors agree—so ask your pediatrician what she recommends. Some say to simply keep the cord dry until it falls off and heals on its own (as in, don't put anything on it; including water). We know of others who recommend dabbing it with alcohol during diaper changes to make it dry up and heal faster—in about 2 weeks, as opposed to the month it could take when left alone. Why the rush? The sooner it heals, the sooner you can give baby a bath in the tub. (You'll have to sponge bathe until then.)

"What the heck am I supposed to do with this penis?"

Take it easy—penises aren't as complicated as they seem. In general, just keep it clean and try to dodge the pee fountains. If your son was circumcised, you'll need to clean the region two or three times a day with warm water (no soap) and apply a lubricant during diaper changes (your pediatrician or hospital should provide one). Also, watch for (rare) signs of infection, like fever, sudden swelling or redness, smelly discharge or pus, or skin that is warm to the touch. (Some of the redness and yellow scabbing is normal and should fade in 7 to 10 days.) After the penis has healed, it's on to basic hygiene. (Clean it with a wipe at diaper changes, and with water in the tub.) If your son still has his foreskin, you don't have to clean under it. (Never try to pull it back before it has separated from the tip of the penis—usually by age 5 or so.) Simply wash on top of it with warm water and gentle soap, the same as you would anywhere else. And don't freak if you see white, pearl-like lumps under the foreskin. This is just the skin cells that shed when the foreskin separates.

"I don't know if I'm burping him right. How am I supposed to do it?"

Burping expels air swallowed during feeding and helps eliminate spit up, crankiness, and gas. Burp when you switch breasts, or after he drinks 2 to 3 ounces. Try these tips:

- Lay baby belly-down on your lap, with his head above his chest, and pat his back.
- Hold baby facing your chest, with his chin on your shoulder. Use one hand to support his head and the other to rub or pat his back. Or, face him outward and leaning a bit forward, supporting his neck and chest with one hand.
- Once baby can hold his head up, you can hold him against your body, facing outward. Gently apply presure on his stomach as you walk around the room.

month 10 ▶

▍in your head

"I wish someone would take this baby away for a few days while I sleep. Does that make me a bad mother?"

No, it makes you normal. Your exhaustion has no implications for your love for your child, or your maternal abilities. Hang in there—it gets better. In the meantime, ask for help. Have someone (your partner? your mom? a friend?) take over baby duty for an afternoon while you sleep between feedings. Also ask someone to go to the grocery store for you, or to cook. Seriously—take advantage of all the help you can get. You deserve it.

"What does postpartum depression feel like? Do I have it?"

Postpartum depression (aka PPD) is a serious illness that affects as many as 20 percent of new moms, causing extreme sadness or anger in the months after baby arrives. If you're one of them, you might feel profoundly sad, hopeless, helpless, irritable, or exhausted, and you might find yourself crying, having trouble eating, or forgetting things. You might also be unable to—or just not want to—take care of yourself and/or the baby. Some women feel better in a few weeks; others suffer for months. If you think you might have PPD, talk to your doctor about treatment options. Luckily, PPD is one of the most treatable forms of depression. Get help, take care of yourself, and everything will be okay. If you're feeling down, isolated, and emotionally fragile just after delivery, it doesn't necessarily mean you have PPD. Lots of moms (as in 70 to 80 percent) also suffer from something called the "baby blues." It's totally normal to feel sad or overwhelmed at first, and to have a good cry now and then. Again, take care of yourself—sleep, eat, and ask for help when you need it. The baby blues usually pass in a few weeks. (If not, or if your symptoms get extreme, talk to your doctor.)

"I still look 5 months pregnant. How long will this last?"

Give your body a break—it just went through a heck of a lot of stretching and strain, and it will take time for it to recover. The good news? Your leftover bump should deflate (for the most part) within a few weeks, as your uterus shrinks back down to its regular plum-size proportions. As for your extra padding, get active as soon as your OB says it's okay, eat right, and you'll start seeing results. Remember, though, that your body went through 9 months of growing and changing. It might take just as long to feel like your old self.

▍is it normal?

"I heard my baby's eyes might change color? When would that happen?"

You heard right. Babies often switch eye colors after birth. Some doctors say it takes between 4 and 6 months to see the true hue, but it's possible for them to change later—even after a year. If you are trying to predict the final color, the biggest clue is your own eye color (and your mate's, of course).

"how did the nurses swaddle my baby so perfectly? I suck at this."

First, cut yourself some slack. Those nurses have had a ton of practice! You'll get the hang of it if you keep trying—here are the basic instructions:

STEP 1 Spread out a lightweight blanket in a diamond shape. Picture a clock face.

STEP 2 Fold the top corner (12 o'clock) down about 6 inches. Place baby's head just above the fold, her feet pointing at 6 o'clock.

STEP 3 Take the right corner (3 o'clock), and wrap it over her right arm and chest. Tuck it behind her back, under her left arm.

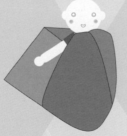

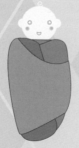

STEP 4 Take the 6 o'clock corner, and pull it up over her feet. Tuck the blanket under her chin.

STEP 5 Pull the final corner (9 o'clock) across her body and around and under her back. Don't be afraid to make it snug.

month 10

"What's up with these first poops?! "

That dark greenish-black, gooey, sticky stuff in his diaper is called meconium, and it's made up of all the stuff baby was swallowing in-utero (amniotic fluid, lanugo, bile, mucus, dead skin cells—yummy).

After a few bowel movements, baby will switch over to mustard yellow poop if you're breastfeeding. It will probably look as though it has seeds in it, and shouldn't smell very bad (score one for nursing!). Breast milk is digested fast, so baby might poop after almost every feeding at first. If you are formula feeding, baby's stool can be yellow, brown, or green, and will smell a little stronger.

See something weird in baby's diaper? If baby's poop is hard and pebble-like, red (could be blood), black (could be digested blood), or white (could signal a liver problem), give the pediatrician a ring. Any other colors are fine.

"Help—my 2-day-old is losing weight! What should I do?"

You should stop freaking out, pronto. Babies can lose up to 10 percent of their birth weight in the first week of life. We repeat, it's *normal*. As long as baby is feeding regularly, peeing, and pooping, he's fine. Most make it back up to their birth weight within 2 weeks.

"I am SO tired, I have a black eye, and my chest hurts. What gives?"

Labor is no picnic. Your body just went through a lot, and it's normal to feel (and see) the strain. And strain, actually, is what probably caused your shiner (you were probably "pushing" with your face during delivery), as well as the achy chest (strained chest muscles, also from pushing). The exhaustion, of course, is par for the course, and you're probably pretty much sore all over. Get as much rest as you can, and report all of your symptoms to your nurse or OB, just to be sure everything is peachy.

"Am I supposed to be bleeding this much? When will it stop?"

Bleeding a lot in the days (and weeks) after delivery is normal. What you're seeing isn't only blood. It's called "lochia" and it contains other leftover stuff from inside your uterus like mucus and tissue. It's likely to be as heavy as your period (remember way back when you had periods?), or even heavier, and it might gush when you stand, or when you breastfeed. This discharge should go from red to pink in the next 3 weeks or so, eventually turning brown, and then a pale yellow or white. Stock up on pads for these next few weeks, and get medical attention immediately if it becomes smelly, turns bright red again after it turns pink or brown, or if you pass a clot bigger than a golf ball (could signal a hemorrhage).

"Why am I sweating through my PJs?"

No one knows for sure, but it's probably your body getting rid of the extra water you've been carrying. (You'll pee a lot of the excess fluids out as well.) Hormones may play a role too, namely the drastic drop in estrogen just after you deliver. This should ease up in a few weeks, but it might last a little longer if you're breastfeeding. It might seem counterintuitive, but staying extra hydrated can help. To keep comfy at night, stash a stack of Ts bedside.

checklist

"what are the absolute essentials I need to care for baby?"

You'll get good use out of all the items in your baby health-care kit, whether you choose to buy an all-in-one set or each product individually.

what you need

○ **THERMOMETER** Buy a digital rectal thermometer. It's as effective as glass, without risk of breaking. You should rely on core temperature for babies, which means ear and forehead thermometers are out for now. Use petroleum jelly to lubricate the thermometer.

○ **NAIL CLIPPERS OR FILE** Babies' nails grow like crazy. Get clippers designed for infants so you don't snip their skin by mistake. If even the miniature clippers seem too scary, stick with filing.

○ **BULB SYRINGE** For tiny noses clogged up with mucus, nasal aspirators are the way to go.

○ **BABY TYLENOL** If your newborn has a fever, call the pediatrician and pay a visit. Docs generally prefer to see such new babies in person.

○ **SALINE** To get dried-up mucus off baby's face.

○ **COTTON SWABS AND BALLS** Moisten these to clean out gooky eyes.

○ **AQUAPHOR** This can be used for all kinds of minor irritations, from dry skin and lips to diaper rash.

○ **BABY COMB/SOFT BRISTLE BRUSH** Especially if your infant has A) hair or B) cradle cap.

○ **GAS DROPS OR GRIPE WATER** Though there's no clinical evidence that these gas remedies work, many parents swear by them. They're benign enough that, if they seem to work for you, use them.

○ **ANTIBIOTIC CREAMS** Talk to your doctor before using Neosporin or other similar topical creams.

month 10

❚ breastfeeding 411

"What if I'm not breastfeeding? Can I make my milk go away?"

If you don't breastfeed, your body will stop making milk. (That's just how it works.) You'll have to go through the engorgement phase first. It will probably hurt, but it shouldn't last more than a day or two. At this time, some moms swear by doubled-up sports bras and other boobie-restricting clothes. Ice packs and pain relievers might help too. Once your breasts have deflated, they might still leak for a few days before drying up.

"I don't think anything is coming out of my boobs when my 2-day-old sucks. Should I give her formula too?"

No, and no. If baby is sucking regularly (every 2 to 3 hours), she is almost definitely getting your colostrum (even if you can't see it). She only needs about a teaspoon's worth at each feeding. Rest assured that your milk should come flooding in on about day 3 or 4. Don't stop now—keep baby breastfeeding regularly to help stimulate your body to fill your boobs.

"I get cramps when I breastfeed— is that supposed to happen?"

When baby sucks, your body makes oxytocin (the same hormone that they use to induce labor). This stuff makes your uterus contract. Why do you need to have contractions now that baby's out? Well, your uterus grew a heck of a lot during pregnancy, and it's on its way back down. The contractions help it shrink. (You can even feel it shrinking by pressing

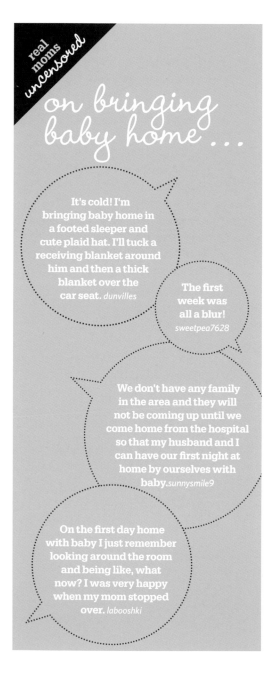

real moms uncensored

on bringing baby home . . .

It's cold! I'm bringing baby home in a footed sleeper and cute plaid hat. I'll tuck a receiving blanket around him and then a thick blanket over the car seat. *dunvilles*

The first week was all a blur! *sweetpea7628*

We don't have any family in the area and they will not be coming up until we come home from the hospital so that my husband and I can have our first night at home by ourselves with baby. *sunnysmile9*

On the first day home with baby I just remember looking around the room and being like, what now? I was very happy when my mom stopped over. *labooshki*

"I'm a wreck about baby's first bath! what do I need?"

Bath time isn't so tough. Once baby's umbilical stump comes off, you can move from sponge baths to "real" baths—in the baby bathtub, in the kitchen sink (make sure it's clean!), or in your arms in the big bathtub (have help getting in and out, and use a non-slip mat). Here's the routine and what you'll need.

washing station Make sure your setup is steady, and position baby's head away from the faucet.

water Fill the tub with about 3 inches of water that's a little bit hotter than lukewarm. Check with your wrist first.

warm room Keep the temperature raised so it's not a shock to baby's system when she comes out of the bath (75 to 80°F).

washcloths Use one color for bath time, another for diaper changes.

plastic cup For rinsing. Or squeeze a wet washcloth over baby's head to get rid of soap.

baby soap A mild, tear-free cleanser for both baby's body and hair is ideal.

extras Remedies that your doctor suggests should be in arms' reach.

how to

Start by soaking baby. Always keep a hand on him (infants are slippery when wet). Start from the top and work your way down. Wash his face first, cleaning one small area at a time. As you move down, thoroughly wash inside all those folds (under the arms, in the neck, the genital area, etc.). Save baby's dirtiest parts (aka the diaper area) for last. Then, move back up and wash baby's hair. Since infants lose most of their heat through their heads, this should be your very last move. If the water is still warm, you can engage in a little playtime, but don't splash for too long—as the water chills, baby will start to get cold.

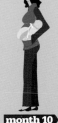

month 10

softly on your tummy.) They can be painful, but the pains should let up within a week. (If they stick around longer, talk to your OB to make sure there's nothing else going on.)

"My breasts are suddenly enormous and they hurt so badly! What do I do?"

On the bright side, congrats—your milk came in! You're engorged, meaning your body just filled your boobs to bursting (don't worry—they won't really burst). It's no fun (at all), but it won't last forever. In the next 24 to 48 hours, your milk supply should level out, and your breasts will soften up. In the meantime, you can relieve the pain by consistently nursing (not pumping) every 2 to 3 hours, even if you have to wake baby for the meal. If your boobs are so rock hard that baby has a tough time latching on, express (by hand or pump) a little milk first to soften things up. While baby sucks, give your boob a nice massage to help the milk keep flowing, and keep baby on one side until it becomes (relatively) soft. Feeding on just one breast per feeding is fine, as long as baby's satisfied. If you're still in pain, try cold packs for a few minutes after feeding, or experiment with the traditional remedy: fresh cabbage leaves. (Rinse them and put them on your boobs.) Whatever you do, don't skip feedings—breastfeeding is a supply-and-demand affair. Not nursing could cause your milk production to take a permanent dip.

> I used the ice packs I got sent home with from the hospital and stuffed them in my bra. I looked funny but hey, it made them feel sooo much better. *mabzie*

"My boobs are leaking constantly. Will this last forever?"

Forever? Probably not. But it can be pretty embarrassing and annoying in the meantime. It's normal in the first weeks of nursing for your breasts to leak, squirt, drip, and spray (fun times). This doesn't happen to everyone, but if you're a leaker, your best defense is to grab some nursing pads and wait. As breastfeeding gets better established, your body won't make more than baby needs, and you'll leak less.

the new day-to-day

"I'm leaking pee. Can I make it stop?"

Do your Kegels! (See page 94.) Lots of women are a little leaky after childbirth, thanks to the loss of muscle tone in the perineum. Kegels can help build the muscles back up, which can help you learn to "hold it" again.

"Will I ever poop again? Will it hurt like hell when I do?"

Yes, you'll poop. If you just delivered, it's normal to take a day or two (or three) to have a bowel movement, usually due to a combo of weak tummy muscles, soreness, and plain old fear. And, to be honest, it might hurt. But probably not as much as you fear. And you won't burst your stitches either. Doing your business just might be a little uncomfortable the first time or two, especially if you have hemorrhoids.

newborn care

cleaning the umbilical cord

During diaper changes, wipe around the area with an alcohol wipe (check with your OB; some think it's better to leave it alone). The remaining cord should fall off in a few weeks. Call your doctor if you see redness, warmth, swelling, or if it still hasn't fallen off in 4 to 6 weeks.

trimming long nails

It's important to keep your baby's nails short so he doesn't scratch his face or eyes. The best way to do this is to trim them with infant-size clippers or file them down while he's sleeping. It might be tempting, but skip the scissors—or biting your newborn's nails.

cleaning out ear wax

Don't stick anything, including Q-tips, into your baby's ear canal, even if you spot wax inside. Eventually, it'll clear out on its own.

bathing

Limit bathing to a few times a week (or as needed). The truth is infants don't get that dirty (exception: very messy poops or spit ups). And until your baby's umbilical cord has fallen off, don't immerse her belly.

changing diapers

Changing them asap is the key to fighting rashes. Girl tip: Wipe front to back to avoid urinary tract infections. Boy tip: It's normal for him to get erections during diaper changes.

To make it easier, eat fiber, drink lots of liquids, take a walk to get your blood flowing . . . and use stool softener if necessary. Plus, try your darndest to relax—tension (in your head and in your butt) definitely won't help matters.

"How long will my c-section cut hurt?"

It will take between 4 and 6 weeks for the incision to heal completely. Constipation can compound the pain, so drink lots of fluids, get up and walk when you can, and pack in the fiber (all of these can help you do a number 2). To further manage pain, use good posture, and hold your tummy when you cough, sneeze, or laugh. If breastfeeding bothers the cut, use a support pillow to get baby off your abdomen. Call your OB if you get a fever over 100.4, start hurting a lot worse, have flu-like symptoms, boob pain, or if your incision turns red, swells, or oozes anything (could be an infection).

"How long will I hurt (down there)?"

Your rate of recovery depends on your physical condition in general and how much labor beat you up, but most moms are feeling a whole lot better by 6 weeks postpartum. (Some sooner, some later.) Every day will get a little better, so try to just take it one achy morning at a time. If you had a tear or episiotomy, speed up healing by keeping your perineum (the tissue between the vagina and rectum) clean and dry. Change sanitary pads every 4 to 6 hours, or whenever you go to the bathroom. Always move from front to back when removing pads or wiping, and wash your hands before and after. These steps prevent bacteria in your stool (yuck!)

from entering your vagina. If it hurts to pee or wipe, use a squirt bottle of warm water to spray the area while you go, and pat dry with gauze when you're done. Witch hazel pads can feel heavenly (line your pad with them), as can a numbing spray like Dermoplast (ask your OB first) and even a few ice cubes in the bathtub. Sitz baths (a few inches of warm water in the tub) are also helpful. Try to take one after every bowel movement. And, don't forget your Kegels—they'll help tighten muscles, improve circulation, and ultimately, reduce the pain. If you have stitches, don't be surprised when pain turns to itching—this is normal as your perineum heals.

"It hurts to sit. I'm too tired to stand."

If it's not practical to lie down all day (don't we all wish it were?), have someone buy you one of those little inflatable doughnut pillows at the nearest drugstore. You'll feel silly, but it'll help because there won't be any pressure.

"When can I have sex again?"

Most new moms get the thumbs up from their health-care providers at around 6 weeks postpartum, depending on the condition of their nether regions. (Are you still bleeding? Have the stitches dissolved?) It takes your uterus and cervix time to heal, even if you had a c-section. When you do get back in the sack, take it slow; it will probably be somewhat uncomfortable the first few times, no matter how you delivered. And if you just aren't ready, that's okay, too—listen to your body and keep communicating with your mate.

diaper bag

size Consider your needs and whether you'll be carrying a regular bag, too. Remember, if there's extra room, you'll fill it.

straps Adjustable straps prevent any slipping. They're also key if more than one person is using the bag.

closure A zipper's ideal for holding everything in. Stay away from Velcro; the ripping noise it makes can wake a sleeping baby.

extra pockets Lots of outer pockets make it quick to find a pacifier, bottle, cell phone, or keys.

base A bag that stands up on its own is easier to reach into.

color If you plan to share, choose a color that suits everyone's taste.

changing pad Make sure it's big enough to be useful—especially as baby grows.

inside the bag

- diapers (one for every two hours, plus a few extra)
- extra changing pad or blanket
- wipes and cream
- important numbers
- extra money
- spare keys
- burp cloths or washcloths
- pacifiers
- bottles and formula
- extra blanket
- change of clothes
- hat
- zipper-top bags
- nursing cover

pregnancy timeline

This handy month-by-month pregnancy guide takes you through every stage of the journey, from week one to delivery.

weeks 1–8
○ Tell your partner
○ Find an OB/GYN
○ Schedule prenatal checkup
○ Make sure partner has short and long term disability
○ Figure out how financials will change
○ Create a savings plan for baby's future expenses
○ Make a budget
○ Have first prenatal checkup (weeks 4–8)

weeks 8–12
○ Buy maternity clothes
○ Chorionic villus sampling
○ Nuchal translucency screening (weeks 10–12)
○ Chromosomal disorder screening (weeks 10–14)
○ Visit the doctor

weeks 12–16
○ Start planning maternity leave and postpartum work schedule
○ Tell boss and loved ones about pregnancy
○ Go to the doctor

weeks 16–20
○ Start planning nursery
○ Look into child care
○ Go to the doctor
○ Have mid-pregnancy ultrasound
○ Amniocentesis and triple screen (weeks 15–18)
○ Find out baby's gender
○ Hear baby's heartbeat
○ Feel first baby kick
○ Notice your growing belly

weeks 20–24
○ Interview pediatricians
○ Research and sign up for childbirth classes
○ If banking cord blood, do research and order kit
○ Visit the doctor

weeks 24–28
○ Update or write will, including inheritance and guardianship info
○ Purchase life insurance
○ Update beneficiaries
○ If using doula and child-care, start interviews
○ Register for shower gifts
○ Go to the doctor

weeks 28–32
○ Start fetal kick counts
○ Prepare birth plan
○ Have your baby shower
○ Send thank-you notes
○ Freeze postpartum meals
○ Start childbirth class
○ Have two doctor visits
○ Others feel baby move

weeks 32–36
○ Buy needed baby items
○ Assemble first aid kit
○ Prep emergency sheets
○ Finish painting nursery
○ Get car seat inspected
○ Pack hospital bag
○ Contact cord blood bank if interested in donating
○ Find out about having additional tests
○ Have two doctor visits
○ Group B strep test (weeks 35–37)
○ Have last day of work
○ Do not fly after week 35

weeks 36–delivery
○ Visit doctor weekly
○ Have non-stress test
○ Get biophysical profile

budget for baby

Here's a list of major purchases and investments over the first year—estimate how much you'll fork over to get a rough answer. And remember . . . the amount you plan to spend doesn't always match the amount you actually do.

one-time expenses:

○ Nursery decorating/ remodeling: _____
○ Crib: _____
○ Crib mattress: _____
○ Bedding and accessories: _____
○ Dresser: _____
○ Rocking chair: _____
○ Changing table: _____
○ Baby monitor: _____
○ Playpen, bouncy chair or walker: _____
○ Safety gates: _____
○ Baby bathtub: _____
○ High chair: _____
○ Bottles: _____
○ Pump: _____
○ Nursing clothes: _____
○ Medicine kit: _____
○ Stroller: _____
○ Baby carrier/sling: _____
○ Car seat: _____
○ Diaper bag: _____
○ Maternity leave salary loss: _____
○ Writing/rewriting will: _____

monthly expenses:

○ Diapers: _____
○ Formula and food: _____
○ Clothes: _____
○ Toys: _____
○ Photo film and developing: _____
○ Extra laundry costs (water, electricity, detergent): _____
○ Child care: _____
○ Life insurance for you and your partner: _____
○ Medical insurance: _____
○ Disability insurance: _____
○ Medical bills (uncovered and co-pays): _____
○ College/education savings: _____
○ Contribution to savings: _____

breastfeeding tracker

baby's name: _____   date: ___ / ___ / ___

feedings

time	breast left	right	feeding duration	baby's mood
:				
:				
:				
:				
:				
:				
:				
:				
:				
:				
:				
:				
:				
:				

diapers

Circle and keep track of baby's diaper changes throughout the day.

pee

poo

time   :   :   :   :   :   :   :   :   :   :

bottle feeding tracker

baby's name: _____   date: _____ / _____ / _____

feedings

time	amount	baby's mood
:	oz.	
:	oz.	
:	oz.	
:	oz.	
:	oz.	
:	oz.	
:	oz.	
:	oz.	
:	oz.	
:	oz.	
:	oz.	
:	oz.	
:	oz.	
	total oz.	

diapers

Circle and keep track of baby's diaper changes throughout the day.

pee

poo

time   :   :   :   :   :   :   :   :   :   :

sleep tracker

**Monitor baby's zzzs. Fill in the date and then
shade in the boxes for hours spent snoozing.**

month: _____

time

date	12 a.m.	2 a.m.	4 a.m.	6 a.m.	8 a.m.	10 a.m.	12 p.m.	2 p.m.	4 p.m.	6 p.m.	8 p.m.	10 p.m.	12 a.m.
1 ___													
2 ___													
3 ___													
4 ___													
5 ___													
6 ___													
7 ___													
8 ___													
9 ___													
10 ___													
11 ___													
12 ___													
13 ___													
14 ___													
15 ___													
16 ___													
17 ___													
18 ___													
19 ___													
20 ___													
21 ___													
22 ___													
23 ___													
24 ___													
25 ___													
26 ___													
27 ___													
28 ___													
29 ___													
30 ___													
31 ___													

need more advice?

American Academy of Pediatrics
Information on physical, mental, and social health from the nation's leading child health experts. **AAP.org**

American College of Nurse-Midwives
Looking for a midwife? Type in your home address and search the national database for a CNM in your area. **ACNM.org**

American College of Obstetrics and Gynecologists (ACOG)
A good place to read up-to-date articles on issues affecting women's health. **ACOG.org**

American Pregnancy Association
In addition to being a strong advocacy group, APA also offers educational articles on sexual health, forums, and will help you find a local health professional. **AmericanPregnancy Association.com**

Association of Women's Health, Obstetric and Neonatal Nurses (AWHONN)
Includes articles from government agencies such as the FDA, CDC and NIH that deal with the latest pregnancy related issues. **AWHONN.org**

Breastfeeding.com
Answers to all of your breastfeeding questions. Plus a supportive breastfeeding community. **Breastfeeding.com**

La Leche League International
Connect with moms in your area and get helpful breastfeeding tips from experienced lactation consultants. **LLLI.org**

Lamaze International
A nonprofit organization that promotes a natural, healthy and safe approach to pregnancy, childbirth, and early parenting. **Lamaze.org**

March of Dimes
Dedicated to improving the health of babies by preventing birth defects, premature birth and infant mortality. **MoDimes.org**

National Center for Fathering
A great resource for dads and dads-to-be looking for advice and more information on their rights as fathers. **Fathers.com**

National Women's Health Resource Center
Features recent health reports, nutritional guides, and a pregnancy and parenting center. **HealthyWomen.org**

National Institute of Child Health and Human Development
Conducts studies on health. Find out about a conference or event that the NICHD may be holding in your area. **NICHD.NIH.gov**

National Organization of Mothers of Twins Clubs
Are you a mommy of multiples? Get connected with other moms in your area who also have twins. **NOMOTC.org**

National Organization of Single Mothers
Focused on helping single mothers cope with the everyday challenges. **SingleMothers.org**

United States Department of Labor
Information and key news about the Family and Medical Leave Act. **DOL.gov/whd/fmla/index.htm**

TheBump.com
The most active mommy community on the Web with the inside scoop on fertility, pregnancy, birth, and everything baby through stage-by-stage advice, interactive tools, and real birth stories.

talk 24/7 on TheBump.com
mom-to-be lingo from TheBump.com/boards

AF Aunt Flo
BC Birth Control
BBT Basal Body Temperature
BD Baby Dance (babymaking sex)
BFP Big Fat Positive (home pregnancy test result)

BF or BF'ing Breastfeeding
IB Implantation Bleeding
LMP Last Menstrual Period
MS Morning Sickness
OWT Old Wives Tale

PCOS, PCOD Polycystic Ovary Syndrome/Disease
PIT Pitocin
US or u/s Ultrasound
VBAC Vaginal birth after cesarian

index

acknowledgments

Congrats, you made it through the whole nine months and beyond. I want to give a great big thanks to all the people who helped create this book:

The million-plus moms on TheBump.com for asking and answering just about every question any mama-to-be could possibly have and new moms everywhere who give us constant inspiration (not to mention practical tips and good advice).

Erin van Vuuren and Paula Kashtan for probing into the wonder of pregnancy and babies to find out every tip, trick, or trend for each month.

The Bump team: Rebecca Dolgin (their fearless leader), Liza Aelion, Melissa Mariola, Kelly Crook, Dawn Camner, Vincent M. Spina, Kate Ward, Kaitlin Stanford, Ellie Martin Cliffe, and Jaimie Dalessio for not even flinching over varicose veins (in the vulva, no less) or vaginal tears, or all the late nights that went into making this book.

My good friend and agent, Chris Tomasino.

My husband, cofounder, and partner, David Liu, and my own babies, Havana, Cairo, and Dublin.

credits

experts

American College of Obstetrics and Gynecologists

Judie Ashworth; Stefanie Weiner
Publicity Managers at Destination Maternity

Shoshana Bennett, Ph.D.
Psychologist, Postpartum Depression Specialist, and Author of *Postpartum Depression for Dummies*

Denise Gershwin, CNM
Certified Nurse-Midwife

Melissa Gould; Ellie Miller
Founding Partners of Ellie & Melissa, The Baby Planners

Kathleen A. Hale, BSN, RN, MS, NE-BC
Associate VP of Nursing at Maine Medical Center

Corky Harvey, MS, RN, IBCLC; Wendy Haldeman, MS, RN, IBCLC
Cofounders and co-owners of The Pump Station & Nurtury

Conner Herman; Kira Ryan
Cofounders of Dream Team Baby

Tricia Higgins
Community Manager at Pampers

Maria Kammerer, CNM
Certified Nurse-Midwife

Erika Lenkert
Author of *The Real Deal Guide to Pregnancy*

Jennifer Loomis
Fine-art Maternity and Family Photographer

Tracy Mallet
Fitness Lifestyle Expert, Author of *Super Fit Mama*

Dr. Vicki Papadeas
Pediatrician at La Guardia Place Pediatrics NYC

Dr. Paula Prezioso
Pediatrician at Pediatric Associates of New York City

Dr. Ashley Roman
Maternal Fetal Medicine Specialist at Maternal Fetal Medicine Associates,

PLLC; Clinical Assistant Professor of Obstetrics and Gynecology at New York University School of Medicine

Sebastiaan Selders
Senior Product Manager at Britax

Andi Silverman
Author of *Mama Knows Breast: A Beginner's Guide to Breastfeeding*

Diane Truong, MD, FAAP; JJ Levenstein, MD, FAAP
Cofounders of MDMoms

Dr. Georgia F. Wortham III MD
Obstetrician at Memphis OB/GYN

moms

Jennifer Beldon, Kristen Case, Jeanine Edwards, Lauren Flanagan, Heather Fleming, Judy Galani-Plasse, Allison Holt, Monica Locksmoe, Julia Lyson, Kari Merkel, Nicole Ragains, Lori Richmond, Alison Salat Bernstein, Lisa Shapiro Dotson, Laura Soloff, Nicole Wertzler

illustration

LULU*/CWC International, Inc., Megan Rojas, Pig Pen Studio

photography

Sonograms courtesy of GE HealthCare; p. 13, 27, 43, 57, 71, 85, 101, 115: Shutterstock; p. 21, from top: Meike Bergmann/Jupiter Images, Klaus Arras/StockFood, Istock Photo, Veer, Photo Alto Photography/Veer, StockFood/Steven Morris Photography, Rita Maas/FoodPix/Getty Images, Food Collection/StockFood; p. 23, 77, 37: Antonis Achilleos; p. 34: Photo Op/StockFood; p. 37, clockwise from top left: Lew Robertson/Corbis, FoodCollection/StockFood (3), Judd Pilossof/StockFood, Shutterstock, FoodCollection/StockFood; p. 38,93: Davies+Starr; p. 49: Gazimal/Stone/Getty Images; p. 65, from top, left to right: Sugar Stock Ltd/Alamy, Stockbyte/Getty Images, Dorling Kindersley/Getty Images, Veronique Leplat/Stockfood Creative/Getty Images, Zabert/Stockfood, Lannretonne/Stockfood, Douglas Johns/Stockfood Creative/Getty Images, Klaus Arras/Stockfood, Laurie Vogt Photography Inc./Stockfood, Crystal Cartier/StockFood Creative/Getty Images, Veer (2), Nicholas Eveleigh/Iconica/Getty Images; p. 78: Mark Lund; p. 89: Ragnar Schmuck/Getty Images; p. 105: Siri Stafford/Digital Vision/Getty Images; p.122, from left: Ellen Silverman, Deborah Jaffe; p. 123, from left: Mark Lund, Martin Poole/The Image Bank/Getty Images; p. 125: Courtesy of Learning Curve Brands Inc.; p. 129: Istock Photo; p. 143: Benjamin Cotton Photographic, Westchester Medical Center; p. 163: Veer.